Ortho ✔ KW-051-427 is
and Management

A GUIDE TO THE CARE
OF ORTHOPAEDIC PATIENTS

Boyd S. Goldie FRCS
Orthopaedic Senior Registrar
Department of Orthopaedic and Traumatic Surgery
The Royal London Hospital
Whitechapel, London

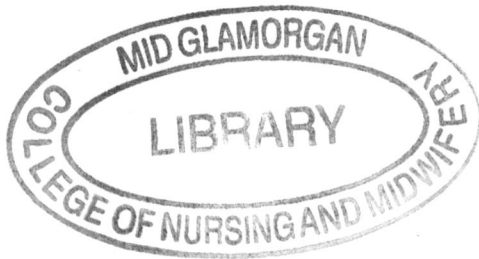

OXFORD

Blackwell Scientific Publications
LONDON EDINBURGH BOSTON
MELBOURNE PARIS BERLIN VIENNA

©1992 by
Blackwell Scientific Publications
Editorial offices:
Osney Mead, Oxford OX2 0EL
25 John Street, London WC1N 2BL
23 Ainslie Place, Edinburgh EH3 6AJ
3 Cambridge Center, Cambridge
    Massachusetts 02142, USA
54 University Street, Carlton
    Victoria 3053, Australia

Other editorial offices:
Arnette SA
2, rue Casimir-Delavigne
75006 Paris
France

Blackwell Wissenschaft
Meinekestrasse 4
D-1000 Berlin 15
Germany

Blackwell MZV
Feldgasse 13
A-1238 Wien
Austria

First published 1992

Set by Excel Typesetters, Hong Kong
Printed and bound in Great Britain
by Hartnolls Ltd, Bodmin, Cornwall

DISTRIBUTORS

Marston Book Services Ltd
PO Box 87
Oxford OX2 0DT
(*Orders*: Tel: 0865 791155
            Fax: 0865 791927
            Telex: 837515)

USA
Blackwell Scientific Publications, Inc.
3 Cambridge Center
Cambridge, MA 02142
(*Orders*: Tel: 800 759–6102)

Canada
Times Mirror Professional Publishing, Ltd
5240 Finch Avenue East
Scarborough, Ontario M1S 5A2
(*Orders*: Tel: 416 298–1588)

Australia
Blackwell Scientific Publications
(Australia) Pty Ltd
54 University Street
Carlton, Victoria 3053
(*Orders*: Tel: 03 347–0300)

British Library
Cataloguing in Publication Data

Goldie, Boyd S.
    Orthopaedic diagnosis
    and management.
    1. Orthopaedics
    I. Title   II. Dunn, David C.
    617. 3

    ISBN 0–632–03043–7

CONSULTANT EDITOR: David C. Dunn

Contents

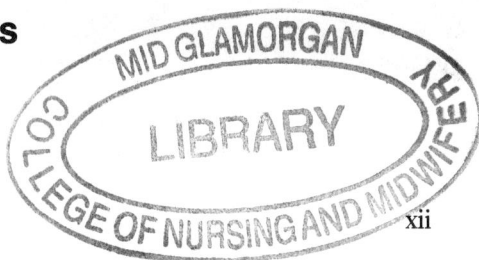

v

Spinal Column

Preface

The stimulus for producing this book came from the repetitive nature of house officers' questions about common orthopaedic conditions and operations. Having used the excellent *Surgical Diagnosis and Management* by David Dunn and Nigel Rawlinson (second edition, 1991, Blackwell Scientific Publications), I decided that the same format could be continued in this book.

The book is designed to be carried in the white coat pocket for rapid reference and aims to answer questions commonly asked by students and junior doctors such as: What is the condition? How do you diagnose the condition? How do you decide when surgery is required? What does the operation entail? What is the management before and after the operation? What complications do you need to know about in order to obtain a proper consent?

In addition, I have tried to give answers to the common questions asked by patients of the doctors: How long will I be in hospital? How long does the operation take? Will I be in a plaster afterwards? When will I be able to go back to work?

I have given what are generally acceptable answers to these questions and I am grateful to the consultants who have carefully checked the text.

This book gives guidance only about orthopaedic surgery. For newly qualified house officers, I strongly recommend that they read the introductory chapters in *Surgical Diagnosis and Management*, since these apply as much to the orthopaedic patient as the general surgical patient.

I hope that this book will make the task of being a junior orthopaedic doctor more fulfilling and less stressful.

Boyd Goldie
The Royal London Hospital

Acknowledgements

I would like to thank Mr David Dunn and Mr John Harrison for their encouragement in bringing this book from an idea into print. I am also grateful to Mr Bill Grange and Mr Marc Patterson for their generosity in taking the time to carefully advise and criticize on the content of the book.

Finally I am indebted to my wife, who has not only put up with the disturbances and absences, but has also had to act as proof reader.

B.S.G.

The layout of this book

After the first chapters on fractures, osteoarthritis, rheumatoid arthritis and complications, subjects are arranged anatomically. Each subject is presented using the standardized headings described below:

The condition
This gives a thumbnail sketch of the condition, with some reference to incidence and aetiology.

Making the diagnosis

The patient
Although there are always exceptions, it is often possible to describe the typical patient who is suffering from a particular condition. Remember that a pattern is being given for ease of identification and that there will always be patients who are atypical.

The history
As in all clinical medicine, the history is the key to most diagnoses. A complete history, including the patient's general health and social history, must not be skimped, even when the radiograph that may have been viewed prior to seeing the patient shows an obvious disorder. I have given certain key points for each condition that will help to keep the history concise.

On examination
I have outlined the most relevant points in the examination. However, certain signs are difficult to describe and are best demonstrated. You should never hesitate to ask your seniors to demonstrate an examination that is unfamiliar to you.

Radiographs
The use of the term X-ray has been avoided since it is medical slang. An X-ray beam is a beam of electro-

magnetic radiation and is invisible. What we look at is the developed film after it has been exposed to the X-rays. This is more properly called a radiograph. Although this may seem pedantic, many surgeons will delight in the opportunity to correct students and junior doctors.

Preoperative management

Investigations
It is assumed that the appropriate investigations for the patient's age, medical history and race will be ordered. Only investigations that are relevant to the orthopaedic condition are mentioned.

Common associated injuries
Patients who have suffered trauma often have injuries that are not immediately apparent at presentation. Always try to consider the possibility of another injury and do not home in on the obvious. One-third of in-patients with a fracture have a second injury that was not diagnosed on admission.

Preparation for surgery

Treatment

Indications for surgery
Certain symptoms and signs must be present as indications for specific operations. If they are absent, the surgery for which the patient has been admitted may be inappropriate and even counterproductive. This is especially true in elective patients who may have been on the waiting list for months (or years) prior to being admitted. In the interval between being placed on the waiting list and admission, they may have completely recovered or deteriorated. If your history and examination makes you question the proposed treatment plan, do not hesitate to inform the surgeon.

Operation

The aim of the description of the procedure is to allow you, the house officer, to understand what is to be done and thus achieve a consent where both doctor and patient are informed!

Codes

The guidance given to you in the codes for each procedure represents what are generally accepted requirements. There is of course a wide variation in the practice of different surgeons and the house officer is advised to note and amend the codes as necessary.

GA/LA. GA, general anaesthetic; LA, local anaesthetic includes spinal, epidural and intravenous regional anaesthetics.

Blood. This is a guide as to how much to crossmatch, and not to the average blood loss. Many blood transfusion departments have policies as to how much blood to make available for common operations, and it is wise to check on this. However, it is the surgical team's responsibility to ensure that an adequate quantity of blood is cross matched, whatever the local guidelines.

Antibiotics. The typical prophylaxis for orthopaedic procedures is three doses of an intravenous antibiotic, usually a cephalosporin, with the first dose given on induction of anaesthesia. Regimes, however, vary from surgeon to surgeon. If you are in doubt, ask.

Time. The time given is only a very rough guide to the length of operation. It is obviously very variable, but it is given because many patients ask how long their operation will take. You should always explain that this is only the operating time and the time between leaving the ward and arriving back is much longer.

Drains. Most orthopaedic surgeons do not suture in the drains. As a general rule, most drainage occurs in the first 24 hours postoperatively. Leaving the drains in longer increases the risk of infection and so drains are usually removed 24 hours after surgery.

Plaster. Most limbs swell following surgery. If plaster

immobilization is required, either a well-padded back-slab or a full plaster that is immediately split, is applied. If a patient has severe postoperative pain, the plaster and dressings must be split down to the skin.

Postoperative radiograph. Bony operations usually require a check radiograph, whereas soft tissue operations do not. The appropriate views have been suggested. The ideal time for taking the radiograph is dealt with under 'Postoperative care' (see below).

Stay. Again only a rough guide to the length of stay postoperatively is given. This is probably the most common question to be asked by patients.

Follow up. The interval between discharge and the first clinic visit depends on whether there are sutures to remove or fractures which need to be closely monitored. If these do not apply, patients are usually seen 6 weeks following surgery. Always ask the surgeon about the time of the follow-up appointment if you are in any doubt.

Off work. The length of time that a patient will be off work depends on their operation and the nature of their work. Remember that many patients with sedentary occupations, who have surgery to their lower limbs, are often off work purely due to their not being able to use public transport.

Operative requirements

Many orthopaedic operations involve specialized equipment. However, the theatre staff may not always know from the title of the operation on the theatre list what is required. Therefore, the theatre staff should be told in advance what is likely to be needed. In addition, the particular equipment should be added to the operating list.

Postoperative care

Management

Much of the guidance given relates to the mobilization of the patient. The surgeon should always state what the regime is to be, so that you, the patient, the nursing staff and the physiotherapists all work to the same plan.

Complications

The complications listed are the complications associated with that particular operation. In a full, informed consent, not only should the orthopaedic risks be mentioned, but also the risks of the anaesthetic and blood transfusion. If you write the headings of the complications that you discuss with the patient on the consent form as you discuss them, you will able to assure a court with greater conviction that they were indeed mentioned.

1   The daily management of patients in orthopaedic wards

Patient records

It is vital that entries are legible, relevant and clearly signed.

Every history sheet must have the patient's name on it in case it becomes separated from the rest of the notes and for medico-legal reasons.

Preoperative check

Each patient should have a check list in the notes with a tick next to each item to indicate that the task has been performed where appropriate and the results of any tests should be given. This list should include the following:

Laboratory tests

Not all patients need the following tests. Refer to *Surgical Diagnosis and Management* (Dunn and Rawlinson, 1991) for guidelines.

FBC U&E }	Write out the blood results in red
CXR	Look at the radiograph yourself and write something to show that you have done so, e.g. lungs clear
ECG	Look at the ECG and make a note, e.g. sinus rhythm
Cross-match	Note the amount

Mark the site and side of operation

To avoid operating on the incorrect side, the operation site should be marked in indelible felt pen with an arrow. The arrow should be drawn prior to the patient receiving their premedication so that you and the patient agree that the correct side is marked.

Do not put the arrow at the site of the incision. For a total hip replacement, an arrow drawn just above the knee, pointing to the appropriate hip, is adequate. For finger and toe operations, the surgeon could potentially operate on the wrong digit. Draw an arrow, indicating the correct digit, on *both* sides of the hand or foot.

In spite of the above, it is ultimately the surgeon's responsibility to check that he is doing the correct operation on the correct patient.

Radiographs   Ensure that the radiographs are on the ward preoperatively and that they accompany the patient to theatre. Once in theatre, put the most recent appropriate radiograph onto the screen.

Consent   The house surgeon usually obtains the consent for surgery from the patient. It is your responsibility to ensure that the description of the operation is accurate, and includes the side and digit where relevant. The writing on the form must be legible, including your signature. Abbreviations must be avoided.

Operating list

In many departments it is the house surgeon's responsibility to write out the routine list that is handed to theatre for typing and distribution. The exact nature of each operation must be given, stating the prosthesis or special equipment that is to be used. Use capital letters and do not use abbreviations, even for the side to be operated upon. The order of the list must be decided by the surgeon. In general, children are put at the beginning of the list, as are diabetic patients. Infected or dirty cases are operated on at the end. Theatres must also be informed if the patient is a potential bio-hazard, e.g. hepatitis B or AIDS. The need for plain radiographs or the image intensifier in theatre must be noted, as a copy of the list is usually sent to the X-ray department. In addition to the above, the house surgeon should always inform the X-ray department, well in advance, if they are likely to be needed.

Tourniquet

It is often the house officer's task to apply the tourniquet. The tourniquet is a pneumatically inflated cuff. The appropriate size of cuff must be chosen relative to the size of the limb. There are a selection of cuffs, from

those small enough for a baby, to that for a large adult
thigh. The use of the wrong size can lead to either
inadequate or excessive compression. Wrap the area
that will be under the tourniquet with a protective
layer of plaster wool. Apply the tourniquet as snugly
as possible and then connect it to the inflation box.
Exsanguinate the limb either by using an Esmarch
bandage or the Rhys Davis exsanguinator. Both of these
require a modicum of skill and you should be shown
how to use them. Whilst the limb is exsanguinated,
inflate the tourniquet to a pressure of 100 mmHg above
the patient's systolic blood pressure. The time of inflation should be noted. The tourniquet is best deflated
after 1½ hours for the upper limb, and 2 hours for the
lower limb.

Operation notes

These are written after each procedure by either the
surgeon or the assistant. They are best written in red to
allow for ease of identification.

In some departments, the surgeon dictates an operation note that is typed and then inserted into the
notes. Since it may take several days for the typed note
to reach the patient's file, it is important that a brief
written note is made in addition.

The information recorded in the operation note
should include the following:

Date.

Title of operation, e.g. cemented Furlong total hip
    replacement.

Surgeon.

Assistant.

Anaesthetist and anaesthetist in charge.

Type of anaesthetic, e.g. GA, LA, Biers, axillary.

Tourniquet time.

Incision/approach, e.g. modified lateral to hip. This is
    important for postoperative mobilization in operations
    around the hip, as patients who have had a posterior
    approach are not generally allowed to sit out of bed as

early as those who have had the lateral or antero-
lateral approach.

Findings. The extent of the handwritten description
depends upon whether or not a note is dictated for
typing. A drawing of an injury or arthroscopic examination can often be helpful.

Procedure. If an implant has been used, record the type
and size. For total hips this includes the size of the
acetabulum, the size of the femoral component, the
neck length and whether or not a cement restrictor
was used. The manufacturer's labels, with the batch
number for each component, must be attached to the
notes.

For a fracture, record the type of plate and the
number of screws inserted.

Closure. Record:
(a) the number and type of drains, e.g. 2 redivacs;
(b) the type of suture to deep layers, e.g. No. 1 Vicryl
to muscle and 2/0 Vicryl to subcutaneous layers;
(c) the type and nature of skin closure, e.g. continuous subcuticular PDS or interrupted nylon.

Postoperative instructions. These are the most important
part of the operation notes. These are the guide for
the nursing staff and the on-call doctor. The instructions should state what particular observations must
be made, mobilization instructions, when the drains
are to be removed and how long antibiotics are to be
continued.

For a routine total hip replacement they may be as
follows:
(a) routine mobilization for posterior approach;
(b) drains out at 24 hours;
(c) AP pelvis on return to ward;
(d) two further doses cefuroxime;
(e) sutures out at 12 days.

Postoperative care of the orthopaedic patient

At the end of the case, the house officer should write up
the antibiotic prophylaxis regime on the prescription

chart and write out the forms for the check haemoglobin and the check radiograph.

On the day of surgery, all patients should have a postoperative check by the duty house officer. This should be recorded in the notes and should include a comment about neuro-vascular function and the amount of drainage.

Subsequent postoperative notes should record whether or not the check radiographs were satisfactory, after what interval the drains were removed, the total drainage during and after surgery, and the postoperative blood results. Each entry must be dated. For ease of reference, the number of postoperative days can be noted at the start of the entry, e.g. 'POD 1' for the first postoperative day.

For any operation where the patient loses a significant amount of blood (for an adult this would be greater than 200 ml), the haemoglobin should be measured on the second postoperative day.

A check radiograph is usually required, with the exception of purely soft tissue operations. In lower limb operations this radiograph is usually obtained before the patient is allowed out of bed. The optimal time to take a check radiograph varies from hospital to hospital. The ideal time (from a surgeon's point of view) is in the recovery room. This allows the surgeon to check the radiograph whilst the patient could potentially be returned to the theatre to correct any disaster. In addition, the patient whilst in recovery still has adequate analgesia. This means that the positioning that is required to take the radiograph is not too distressing for the patient. Radiographs taken in recovery require considerable co-operation from the X-ray department.

In some hospitals, the patient returns to the ward via the X-ray department. This occupies a recovery nurse for an additional length of time and it may not be ideal for a patient who has undergone a major operation to be in the X-ray department. For major cases (e.g. total hip replacement), it may be best to wait until the second postoperative day to take the check radiograph, as the patient may find the positioning very uncomfortable.

Ward rounds

A note should be made for all rounds, including whose round it was and exactly what policy decisions were made. An entry should be made at least daily, for all postoperative patients. Even for long stay patients, an attempt should be made to see each patient and record a note daily. There is no excuse for lack of entries in the notes, and the coroner will ask for an explanation if a patient dies with inadequate notes.

For consultant ward rounds there are several hints to ensure that things run smoothly.

1 Present the patient concisely, mentioning the patient's name, age, diagnosis (including the side) and length of time postoperatively. If you have problems remembering who has had what and when, write a list of the patients in the order that they are to be seen.

2 Organize the radiographs prior to the ward round. If the patient is due to have an operation, have the most recent relevant radiographs at the front of the packet. If the patient had a fracture that has been treated, have the immediate preoperative and the recent postoperative radiographs to hand. There is nothing worse than watching the house officer struggle with a pile of radiographs which seem to have a mind of their own.

3 Become acquainted with the correct orientation of radiographs — if in doubt ask.

2 Fractures

The condition

A fracture is a break in continuity of a bone. There is no difference between a break and a fracture (as many patients suppose).

A fracture may be closed or open. A compound fracture is the same as an open fracture.

Making the diagnosis

The patient

Certain fractures occur more commonly in certain patients. The main variable is age. For example, a fall onto the outstretched hand commonly results in the following:

Toddler	Greenstick fracture of the distal radius
Infant	Injury to the distal radial epiphysis
10–15 years	Fractured clavicle
Young adult	Scaphoid fracture
Middle aged	Colles' fracture
Elderly	

The history

The symptoms of a fracture are pain and loss of function. The intensity of the pain may vary in different patients with similar fractures. Do not be dissuaded from asking for a radiograph if the patient only has minimal pain if you otherwise think that there could be a fracture. Remember that pain may be referred. Pain in the knee for example, may be due to an injury to the hip.

The loss of function associated with a fracture may be complete, e.g. being unable to weight bear with a tibial fracture. There may be only partial loss of function, such as pain on using the wrist with a scaphoid fracture.

Always ask about loss of power or abnormal sensation distal to the fracture. This may indicate a nerve or vessel injury associated with the fracture.

When taking the history, you must ascertain when the injury occurred and in what environment (very import-

7

ant if it is an open fracture). Try and establish the exact mechanism of injury. Simply knowing that the patient was playing football is not enough. The attitude of the hand when falling will often predict the type or configuration of the fracture.

Enquire about any symptoms away from the obviously broken bone, in particular, the adjacent joints.

If the upper limb is injured, ask the patient if they are right or left handed.

Always take a social history. Treatment of the fracture may be influenced by the occupation of the patient. For example, a metacarpal fracture in the left hand of a professional violinist might need internal fixation whereas that of a psychiatrist may not! Any patient, of any age, who lives alone is severely handicapped by a cast. Ensure that the patient will be able to look after themself if they are sent home with a leg or arm in a plaster cast.

On examination   If the patient has had a high energy injury, such as a car accident or falling from a height, examine the whole patient as fractures are commonly missed.

The following classical signs of a fracture may or may not be present:

Deformity. Deformity may be gross or subtle.

Swelling. Fracture of a bone is usually associated with a varying degree of soft tissue swelling. If there is massive swelling, there may also be fracture blisters. It is important that you note the presence of these blisters, as they can get infected.

Tenderness. Gently examine the patient to determine the *exact* site of tenderness.

Crepitus. This grating of the two ends of the bones should not be deliberately elicited.

Try and examine the adjacent joints. Obviously you cannot test the range of movement of the knee with an unstable tibial fracture, but you can look for swelling, bruising and tenderness.

Note any wound or soft tissue damage.

Check on the integrity of neuro-vascular function distal to the fracture. Essentially this means palpating the pulses, checking sensation and asking the patient to move their fingers or toes.

Radiographs   Radiographs in two planes must include the whole bone and the adjacent joints.

When describing a fracture on a radiograph (often by telephone) state the following:

1 Which bone.

2 Which side, left or right.

3 What part of the bone. For long bones, consider the bones in thirds, e.g. the fracture may be in the distal third or at the junction of the middle and distal thirds.

4 Is the fracture intra-articular? If the fracture is near a joint, does it extend into that joint?

5 Is the adjacent joint intact? Or is there a subluxation or dislocation?

6 What is the configuration of the fracture? Are there two or three major fragments, or is the fracture comminuted? Is the fracture transverse, oblique, spiral? Is there a butterfly fragment? If the fracture is due to the pull of a tendon, the fragment may look as if it has been avulsed.

7 The displacement. Displacement must be described for each of the two planes of the radiographs. Displacement may be:

(a) sideways shift or translocation — if so estimate the amount in relation to the width of the bone (e.g. shifted by 50% of the width of the cortex on the AP view);

(b) angulation — describe the distal fragment in relation to the proximal;

(c) torsion — this is usually more obvious clinically, but an AP view of the knee with a lateral view of the ankle on a single radiograph implies considerable rotation.

Preoperative management

Investigations   Some fractures need more than just plain radiographs. Tomograms or CT scans are commonly required for spinal fractures.

Common associated injuries

Nerves, vessels and tendons can all be injured.

Treatment

Fractures that are displaced may need to be reduced. The reasons for reducing a fracture include:

Improving the function after the fracture has united.

To increase the chance of union of the fracture.

To minimize the risk of late arthritis if the fracutre is adjacent to a joint or intra-articular.

Cosmesis.

The fracture can be reduced by manipulation, traction or open reduction. Once reduced, the position needs to be maintained. There are several ways of achieving this.

Anatomy of fracture

Some fractures are inherently stable and do not require additional stabilization.

Plaster cast

The position may be held by a cast that includes both the adjacent joints if the fracture is in the middle of a bone, or only the nearby joint if the fracture is at the end of a bone.

External fixator

If the fracture is open, the position is usually held with an external fixator. This method allows wound management whilst holding the fracture reduced (see Chapter 3). External fixators may be used for closed fractures if the comminution precludes successful treatment by either an external cast or internal fixation.

Traction

Fractures may be reduced and/or held by traction. Traction may be by skin traction, where adhesive tape is stuck to the limb distal to the fracture and weights applied. Skin traction is limited by the amount of weight

that·can be applied before the skin is damaged. Two
and a quarter kilograms (5 lbs) is generally safe. Skin
traction is used on children as the definitive form of
traction for hip and femoral fractures. In the elderly,
skin traction is applied as a means of temporary immobilization in patients with a femoral neck fracture.
Skeletal traction is applied via a pin inserted into or
through the bone. The advantages of skeletal traction
over skin traction are that the weight that can be applied
is much greater and traction can be continued for
longer.

Internal fixation
Fractures can be internally fixed after reduction by
either plates and screws applied to the bone, or by
devices that pass down the medullary cavity of a long
bone. The advantages of successful internal fixation are
two-fold. First, the accurate reduction of intra-articular
fractures minimizes the risk of degenerative change in
the joint. Secondly, a strong stable fixation allows early
return of function of the limb. The disadvantages of
internal fixation are the risk of infection and of not
achieving the aim of a stable strong reduction that goes
on to solid union.

Applying a plaster

Many hospitals employ a plaster technician who applies
plasters for the casualty department and the fracture
clinic. A technician is not usually present at night or in
theatre and the house officer is often required to apply
back-slabs and full plasters. Take every opportunity to
learn how to apply a plaster from the plaster technician
and from the registrars and consultants.

There are several tips that may make your plastering
easier:
1 If the limb has *not* been operated upon, you can put a
Tubinet bandage on the limb first. Make sure that it is
not too tight and do not use Tubigrip. Apply plaster
wool smoothly over the Tubinet. Remember that any

bumps may become areas of high pressure and result in pressure sores under the plaster.

2 Plaster of Paris sets by an exothermic reaction and thus gets hot. If hot water is used to wet the plaster, the already hot water is further heated and it is possible to burn the patient. Therefore use cool or tepid water. This also slows the rate at which the plaster sets and gives you more time to apply the cast.

3 Remember that any indentation that is made in the plaster as it is setting will remain and can cause a pressure sore. When holding a limb that is being plastered, try to hold it by parts that are not being included in the plaster, e.g. the toes and above the knee for a below-knee plaster. If this is not possible, support the limb with the palm of the hand rather than the fingertips. Always hold the limb in the position in which it is to remain. In other words do not bend an elbow or a knee after applying the wool or the plaster, as the wool and plaster may cause neuro-vascular compression.

4 If the plaster is being applied to an acutely injured limb or one which has been operated upon, there is a risk of swelling. In this case, either put on a back-slab, or a full plaster that is split longitudinally.

5 Fibreglass casting material should not be used by the inexperienced, as it is difficult to use and quite unforgiving.

6 Learn how to use the plaster saw and the implements for removing a plaster. The blade of the plaster saw does not rotate, but oscillates. In theory, if the blade touches the skin, it will not cut it. Always explain this to patients, who are naturally apprehensive when first confronted with the plaster saw. Remember not to drag the blade down the plaster but to use repeated downward cuts. Try to use different parts of the blade, as it can become quite hot.

Removal of K-wires and traction pins

It is often the house officer's task to remove K-wires and traction pins from patients on the ward. Both wires and pins can be removed without local anaesthetic from adults. This should be done in a clean area, such as the treatment room. It is often best to give the patient an analgesic prior to the pin extraction. Tell the nursing staff when you intend to remove the pin, so that they can give the analgesic in good time.

For a K-wire that is protruding through the skin, you will need a large needle holder or some pliers, gloves, antiseptic solution and a small dressing pack containing gauze, forceps and a small receptacle. Look at the position of the pin on the radiograph and work out in which direction you have to pull. Thoroughly clean the pin and the surrounding skin. Firmly grasp the pin, twist it and pull hard. If the wire does not come out easily, try one more time to remove it before asking the advice of a more senior person.

Femoral and tibial traction pins pass completely through the leg and it is important not to draw infection into the bone when the pin is removed. You need a dressing pack, antiseptic solution, gloves and a 'Jacob's chuck and key'. Look at the radiograph to see if the pin has threads in the middle. Alternatively, look in the notes to see if the pin is a Denham pin, which is threaded, or a Steinmann pin, which is smooth. Thoroughly clean the pin, removing all congealed blood and debris from the side of the pin that is to pass through the bone. Remove the pin using the Jacob's chuck and put dressings over the holes. If the holes ooze a lot, wrap the leg with plaster wool and a crepe bandage.

3   Open fractures

The condition

An open (compound) fracture is a fracture associated with a break in the overlying skin. The break in the skin may be due to the broken bone coming out, or due to the external impact that resulted in the fracture. Open fractures have a great risk of becoming infected and the risk increases with the size of the wound. Open fractures are graded as follows:

Type I   A skin wound less than 1 cm that is clean

Type II   A laceration more than 1 cm long, without extensive soft tissue damage, flaps or avulsions

Type III   A large severe wound with extensive skin and soft tissue contusion, muscle crush or loss. This grade is subdivided into;

III(a) adequate soft tissue cover of the fractured bone despite extensive soft-tissue laceration or flaps

III(b) extensive soft tissue loss with periosteal stripping and bony exposure

III(c) an open fracture associated with an arterial injury requiring repair, irrespective of the degree of soft tissue injury

Preparation for surgery

Preoperative management

Cultures should be taken from the wound and then the wound must be covered with a sterile dressing. Once covered, the wound should remain undisturbed until the patient reaches theatre.

Indications for surgery

Treatment

All open wounds need debridement and irrigation within *6 hours* of the time the accident occurred and not 6 hours of arriving in casualty. The fracture has to be reduced and then immobilized.

14

Operation: irrigation and debridement of an open fracture

All contaminated and devitalized tissue is excised. If necessary the wound may be extended to allow access to the damaged muscle. The wound is irrigated with copious amounts of saline. The wound is not closed with the exception of a type I injury that is completely clean. In general, the wound is packed and the fracture is immobilized either in a plaster, by traction, or by an external fixator. Secondary closure is performed if the wound is clean when inspected after 48 hours.

Codes

GA/LA	GA
Blood	Appropriate to fracture
Antibiotics	Yes
Time	Depends on wound
Drains	0
Plaster	Yes
Postoperative radiograph	Yes

Operative requirements

A tourniquet should be placed, but only used if unavoidable.

Postoperative care

Management

If the wound is left open, the patient will have to return to the theatre after 48 hours. Antibiotics should be continued until the wound is closed.

If the skin loss has been considerable, the wound may need to be covered with a split thickness skin graft or a local muscle flap.

If the wound is clean after 48 hours, internal fixation may be performed and the wound closed.

Complications

Wound infection.
Osteomyelitis.

It is not the role of the house officer to direct the initial management of the patient with multiple injuries. However, you will be involved and several things should be remembered.

Airway
Ensure that the patient has an airway that is clear and not blocked by dentures, tongue or vomit.

Breathing
If the patient is not breathing, you should not attempt to intubate the patient unless you have considerable experience. A properly applied face mask is usually adequate.

Intravenous access
Use a cannula through which blood can be given. The smallest acceptable is a 16 gauge, but a 14 gauge is preferred. Insert two cannulae if possible. Take blood for cross-match, full blood count and biochemistry when you insert the cannula.

Cross-match
If there is a significant injury, order blood to be cross matched and not just grouped and saved. If there is more than one injury, order enough blood. It is easy to underestimate what may be lost. If in doubt ask the senior person how much should be cross matched.

Radiographs
The minimum that is required is a lateral view of the whole of the cervical spine, a chest radiograph, and an AP of the pelvis. These should be taken in the resuscitation room using the portable X-ray machine. Radiographs of an obviously fractured limb are not essential in the initial period of resuscitation.

Rheumatoid arthritis

The condition

This is a common disease that usually presents in middle age and in women more than men. It is a systemic inflammatory disease that primarily affects synovial joints. It can affect most joints, both large and small.

Making the diagnosis

The patient

By the time a patient with rheumatoid arthritis presents to the orthopaedic department, the diagnosis is usually established.

The history

The rheumatoid patient often has an extensive medical and surgical history. However, there are several parts of the history that must be elicited.

How long has the patient had the disease and is it active or quiescent (burnt out)?

How mobile is the patient and which joints most limit the patient's activities?

Which joint is most painful?

For all the major joints, first ask about pain and stiffness in the joint. Secondly, in your past surgical history ask about operations to each joint. Try to include all procedures, in chronological order for each separate joint. The joints to be considered are shoulders, elbows, wrist, hands, hips, knees, ankles and feet.

Always ask if the patient has any neck pain, since rheumatoid arthritis can lead to instability of the cervical spine. The disease can also affect the temporo-mandibular joints and make them stiff. Both of these points are important in regard to anaesthesia. Excessive movement of an unstable neck during intubation can injure the spinal cord and intubation itself may be very difficult if the mouth cannot be opened due to stiffness of the temporo-mandibular joints.

Take a drug history that includes past intra-articular steroid injections. Also find out if the patient is currently taking systemic steroids. If they are, the patient may require additional steroids in the perioperative period.

Take a careful social history. Does the patient live alone? If so, they may need additional social services once discharged from hospital. Do they have stairs to climb? If so, how many?

On examination

In a severe rheumatoid, a complete examination is a formidable task. It is best to be methodical and examine each joint in turn. Tabulate the findings in two columns, left and right. Place the 'right' column on the left, and the 'left' column on the right. This is easier to fill in, as this is the way that you look at the patient.

For each major joint, note any swelling, deformity, instability, range of movement and whether movement is painful throughout the range of movement or just at the end of the movement.

Radiographs

The signs of rheumatoid arthritis begin with diffuse porosis of the bones on both sides of the joint. The joint space becomes narrowed and finally the joint is destroyed. The joint may become subluxed or even dislocated.

Try to be selective in your request for radiographs. Check the patient's packet to see when radiographs were last taken of the symptomatic joints. In general, new views are only required if the interval is greater than 6 months, or if there has been a marked clinical deterioration since the last radiographs were taken. Always ensure that there are views of the cervical spine.

Preoperative management

Investigations

Rheumatoid patients are often anaemic and have a raised erythrocyte sedimentation rate. Although often requested, the serological tests for rheumatoid arthritis are not very helpful in either diagnosis or treatment.

Treatment

The role of the physiotherapists, occupational therapists, social workers and nurses should not be underestimated in this debilitating, destructive disease.

The initial treatment is always conservative. This includes resting a joint that is acutely inflamed either by bed rest or splints. In the non-inflamed state, joints are kept mobile with physiotherapy and home exercises.

Systemic treatment is usually supervised by the rheumatologists. The choice of anti-inflammatory ranges from aspirin, to non-steroidal anti-inflammatory drugs, to systemic steroids. Other drugs, such as gold, are also used. Steroids can be injected directly into an inflamed area and give good relief of pain. However, the injections cannot be given more than twice into any one site as there are risks of tendon rupture.

Indications for surgery

The main indication for surgery is pain. Joint stiffness alone is *not* an indication for surgery. Indeed a stiff but pain-free joint is a contra-indication to surgery and is the aim of an arthrodesis. Surgery may be indicated to correct deformity and improve function:

Synovectomy, removal of the diseased synovium, is effective in some joints in reducing pain and slowing down joint destruction. Synovectomy around the tendon sheaths may prevent tendon rupture.

Repair of ruptured tendons and soft tissue correction of deformities (especially in the hands), may considerably improve function.

Arthrodesis (fusion) of some joints may improve function in the adjacent joints by providing stability and reducing pain. Wrist fusion is a good example.

Joint replacement has a major role in the surgical treatment of rheumatoid arthritis. The relief of pain is predictable and the joints perform well. This is because the patients are less active than those with osteoarthritis. However, the risk of infection is higher in rheumatoid patients, especially if they are on systemic steroids.

The condition

Osteoarthritis is the result of degeneration of the articular cartilage of a joint. If there is no known precipitating cause for the degeneration, then the osteoarthritis is considered to be primary. In most cases there is an identifiable cause for osteoarthritis. There may be an abnormality within the joint, such as previous intraarticular fracture or removal of the meniscus of the knee. Alternatively, there may be abnormal stresses through the joint — either excessive as in obesity, or repetitive as in high level sportsmen, or in an abnormal direction, such as following a fracture which has healed in an abnormal alignment.

Making the diagnosis

The patient

Most patients with osteoarthritis of a joint do not present until after middle age. However, if the degeneration follows a childhood problem (e.g. congenital dislocation of the hip), presentation may be as early as the second decade.

The history

You must take a careful history that extends as far back as the patient can recall. Patients often dismiss previous injuries as irrelevant if they occurred a long time in the past. Always enquire about the patient's previous occupation and hobbies. Ask about previous surgery to the limb.

As with any pain, ask about the site, nature, intensity, character, relieving factors, exacerbating factors and radiation. Assess the function of the joint by establishing how limited the patient is in his/her daily activities.

On examination

Look at the limb and the joint. Is there any deformity, muscle wasting or scarring? If the joint is enlarged, palpate the joint and decide if any swelling is bony due to osteophytes, or non-bony due to an effusion. Test the stability of the joint to see if the ligaments are intact. Establish the range of movement, both actively and passively. Is there a fixed deformity (that does not vary with the position of the joint) and is there crepitus on moving the joint? Is the joint purely stiff, or does movement of the joint cause pain?

Radiographs   The first sign of osteoarthritis, loss of joint 'space', reflects the fact that it is loss of articular cartilage that is the main pathology. This joint space which is lost is, of course, the radiolucent articular cartilage. The later changes are osteophyte formation around the periphery of the joint, subchondral bone sclerosis (looks very white on the radiograph) and cyst formation.

Treatment

Conservative treatment should always be considered before surgery. Weight loss, change in occupation, use of a walking stick, mild analgesics and anti-inflammatories can all be effective. Physiotherapy may be useful in both relieving pain and increasing the range of movement.

The aim of surgery is primarily to relieve pain. Any gain in movement is purely an added bonus. A stiff but painless joint is a contra-indication to surgery. Surgical treatment includes arthrodesis, osteotomy and arthroplasty:

Arthrodesis aims to produce a joint that is completely stiff, but pain free.

Osteotomy realigns load transfer through a joint. The mechanism behind the success of osteotomies has not been completely explained but they can provide long lasting pain relief. Neither arthrodesis nor osteotomy precludes later conversion to an arthroplasty.

Joint replacement is not possible for all joints and not ideal in the younger patients. There are major risks in the replacement of joints including infection, intra-operative and late bone fracture, failure of the components themselves and loosening of the components. Revision (reoperation) of joint replacement is always more difficult than the original operation and the results less predictable. However, when performed for the correct indications, joint replacement can transform a patient's life.

One of the most serious complications following an orthopaedic operation is deep infection. The presence of a foreign body, even though sterile when inserted, acts as a nidus for infection. Once there is deep sepsis, the only way of removing the infection may be to remove the prosthesis.

The most common organism which infects prostheses is *Staphylococcus aureus*. However, *Staphylococcus epidermidis*, although regarded generally as non-pathogenic, can also cause deep infection.

In elective cases, where a prosthesis is to be inserted, the following measures should be taken:

1 On admission send a sample of midstream urine to microbiology for microscopy, culture and sensitivity. If the patient has a urinary tract infection, this should be treated prior to surgery.

2 The patient is given a bath or shower using an antiseptic soap, on the night before and on the day of surgery.

3 The operation is performed in a dedicated orthopaedic theatre. In many hospitals, the orthopaedic theatre has an ultra-clean air system of one sort or another. In some units the surgeon and assistants may operate wearing an exhaust suit that looks like a space suit. It is designed to carry away air from the surgeon's (dirty) body out of the operating field.

4 Because orthopaedic surgeons handle bone that has sharp and spiky edges, they usually operate wearing two pairs of gloves. This precaution means that if the outer glove is unknowingly perforated, the inner will prevent possible contamination from the surgeon's skin. After prepping and draping the patient on the operating table, it is best to change the outer gloves, as they may have become contaminated. When the prosthesis itself is inserted, the surgeon changes his gloves for a new pair, in case he has unknowingly contaminated the first.

If at any time you feel that either you or the surgeon may have desterilized their gloves or gown, or an instrument or drape has become contaminated, you *must* inform the surgeon. No one will criticize you for trying to avert a disaster.

5 Whenever a prosthesis is inserted patients *must* receive antibiotic prophylaxis. Prostheses include artificial joints, both metal and plastic, screws, plates and intramedullary nails. Temporary K-wires do not need antibiotic cover. The commonest regime for prophylaxis is three intravenous doses of a second generation cephalosporin, such as cefuroxime. The first dose must be given with induction of anaesthesia prior to the inflation of a tourniquet. If the patient is truly allergic to penicillin you can give a test dose of the cephalosporin to see if the patient is also allergic to that as well. If a cephalosporin cannot be used, give the patient three intravenous doses of erythromycin.

6 Whenever a patient who has had a prosthesis inserted undergoes any further procedure that may result in a bacteraemia, they *must* be given antibiotic cover. If the patient requires a urinary catheter, prescribe oral trimethoprim whilst the catheter is in situ. Tell the patient that should they have any dental procedure, they need to receive antibiotic prophylaxis and they should inform their dentist.

In trauma cases undergoing surgery, preoperative urine sample and antiseptic wash is often not possible, but the surgical techniques remain the same. For a closed fracture, the three dose cephalosporin regime is adequate. In open injuries, swabs should be taken from the wound and antibiotic therapy continued for a minimum of 48 hours (see Chapters 3 and 36).

Tetanus prophylaxis

In all patients with a wound, check that the patient is covered against tetanus:

1 A patient who has active immunity and received their last dose of tetanus toxoid within the last 5 years needs no further prophylaxis.

2 A patient whose last dose of toxoid was greater than 5 years ago should be given a tetanus toxoid booster.

3 A patient who has never completed a tetanus toxoid course should commence one.

8

Compartment syndrome

The condition

A compartment syndrome occurs when high pressure within a closed fascial space reduces capillary perfusion below a level necessary for tissue viability. Intracompartmental pressure may become raised due to interstitial oedema, haemorrhage or muscle fibre swelling within the compartment. Compartment pressure may also become elevated by external constriction of the compartment (e.g. tight casts).

If a compartment syndrome is not effectively treated, the muscle within the compartment dies and fibroses. This results in a Volkmann's ischaemic contracture.

Making the diagnosis

The patient
The patient may be acutely injured, having suffered a blow or crushing injury. Although a fracture may be present, it is the soft tissue injury that is important. Alternatively, the patient may be at risk following an operation which involved considerable soft tissue trauma or was performed under a pneumatic tourniquet.

The history
The cardinal feature of a compartment syndrome is increasing pain, unrelieved by increased doses of analgesics. Later when the nerve that runs through the compartment becomes ischaemic, there will be paraesthesia and then numbness in the distribution of that nerve.

On examination
Stretching the muscles that are involved in the compartment syndrome increases the pain. When examining a patient who is at risk from a compartment syndrome, you must be gentle but thorough. In the upper limb with a forearm fracture, moving the fingers to a new position may be painful even without a compartment syndrome. What is significant, is if the discomfort/pain continues when the fingers are held extended without further movement. Likewise with the toes.

Since the major vessels have a greater pulse pressure than the microvascular circulation that is being compressed, one may find a palpable radial pulse at the wrist in the presence of a compartment syndrome. In short, the presence of a distal pulse does not exclude a compartment syndrome.

Examine the muscles of the leg or arm. In compartment syndrome, they may feel abnormally firm, and direct pressure is painful.

Examine sensation in the hand or the foot.

Preoperative management

Investigations

The pressure in a compartment can be measured. However, lack of a means of measuring the compartment pressure should not detract from the clinical diagnosis and the need to operate.

Measurement can be done under local anaesthetic in casualty. The compartment pressure can be measured using a sphygmomanometer, a three way tap and a saline column as used for measuring the central venous pressure. This is the Whiteside technique. Alternatively, there are hand-held devices which have a needle which is inserted into the compartment and which display the pressure in the compartment on an electronic readout.

In the forearm, the pressure in the deep and superficial compartments has to be measured. In the lower leg the pressure in all four compartments, the superficial posterior, the deep posterior, the anterior and the lateral, must be measured. If the compartment pressure is greater than the diastolic blood pressure minus 30 mmHg, then a compartment syndrome is likely.

Treatment

Indications for surgery

Clinical suspicion of a compartment syndrome.

Operation: decompressive fasciotomy for compartment syndrome

A true compartment syndrome is an emergency and time is of the essence.

In the forearm, a long curvilinear incision is made from the antecubital fossa down the radial side of the flexor muscles and across the wrist. The skin and all layers of the fascia are divided.

In the leg, the incisions depend upon which compartments are involved. The superficial and deep posterior compartments can be decompressed through a long posterior stocking-seam incision. The anterior and the lateral compartments can be reached through a single antero-lateral incision. Some surgeons prefer to decompress all four compartments through the single lateral incision.

In a true compartment syndrome, the muscle will bulge out through the fascia as it is cut and will look bruised and dusky. If there is a concomitant fracture, it is best fixed internally or stabilized with an external fixator. The open wound is dressed. The patient will have to return to theatre for delayed closure of the wound once the muscle swelling has subsided. Complete closure of the skin is often impossible even after 10 days and the defect may need to be covered with a split skin graft.

Codes

GA/LA	GA . . . .
Blood	Group and save . . . .
Antibiotics	Yes . . . .
Time	30 minutes . . . .
Drains	0 . . . .
Plaster	Yes . . . .
Stay	10 days . . . .
Follow up	2 weeks . . . .
Off work	6 weeks minimum . . . .

Operative requirements   No tourniquet.

Management

Postoperative care
Gentle elevation of the limb.
Continue antibiotics whilst the wound remains open.

Complications   Wound infection.

Incomplete fasciotomy resulting in a degree of late contracture.

9   Deep venous thrombosis

The condition

Deep vein thrombosis is a common complication in orthopaedic patients. Most thromboses are subclinical and the diagnosis may only be made retrospectively with the appearance of the signs of venous incompetence. In operations around the hip, at least a third of patients develop a deep venous thrombosis, but only a minority become symptomatic. The thrombosis usually develops during surgery, but you must remember that many patients awaiting elective surgery are very inactive and may develop a thrombosis preoperatively.

Making the diagnosis

The patient

The patient at risk is a patient of any age who is themselves immobilized or has the lower limb immobilized or has had an operation on the lower limb. Classically the presentation is 7–10 days postoperatively.

The history

Most deep vein thromboses are pain free and clinically 'silent'. The patient may complain of calf pain. There may be a slight pyrexia and a mild tachycardia.

On examination

The signs depend upon whether the thrombosis is confined to below the knee, or extends above the knee. A patient with a below-knee thrombosis will have calf tenderness and increased pain on dorsiflexion of the ankle. The calf may be measurably swollen. Acute thrombosis of the femoral or iliac veins leads to a grossly swollen leg and localized tenderness over the involved vein. The difficulty is in distinguishing the mild oedema that occurs after any leg operation from the swelling associated with a deep vein thrombosis. The two indicators of the latter are the pain and the time interval.

Management

Investigations

Patients at risk for developing a thrombosis can be screened using radioactive labelled fibrinogen, which is injected intravenously. A Geiger counter is used to make daily counts at predetermined levels in the limb. A localized increased uptake of fibrinogen may indicate a thrombosis and the patient should then have a venogram. This technique of screening with labelled fibrinogen is mainly used as a research technique.

If a patient clinically has a thrombosis, the veins can be examined using the portable Doppler ultrasound probe. The probe is placed over the popliteal vein and the femoral vein. Phasic flow in time with the respiration is normal and indicates that the vessel is patent. Squeezing the calf should produce a whoosh of flow if the veins are patent. If only high pitched, non-phasic flow is heard, this may indicate early collateral venous flow. Alternatively, no flow may be heard. The Doppler is 90% accurate in the diagnosis of femoral thrombosis and above, but not so accurate below the popliteal fossa.

The definitive investigation for a suspected deep vein thrombosis is the venogram. Radio-opaque contrast is injected into a vein in the foot and the venous tree is imaged. If a femoral thrombosis is suspected, you must specifically request that the upper end of the clot is seen. This is because a clot extending into the iliac veins has a high risk of detaching and causing a pulmonary embolus. Some vascular surgeons recommend the insertion of an 'umbrella' in the inferior vena cava in this situation.

Prophylaxis

The policies for prophylaxis against deep vein thrombosis vary widely. The difficulty is in deciding who should receive prophylaxis and by what means.

The at-risk population includes anyone having lower limb surgery or hip surgery, patients on bed rest and patients who have a plaster cast on the leg.

The intraoperative prophylactic measures include a TED (thromboembolic deterrent) stocking on the unoperated leg or both legs, pneumatic boots, electrical calf stimulators and intravenous dextran. Postoperatively patients can wear TED stockings, be given subcutaneous heparin 5000 units b.d., be fully heparinized or warfarinized, or be given low dose warfarin maintaining a prothrombin ratio between 1.5 and 2.

In short it is best to find out the policy of your consultant for who receives deep vein thrombosis prophylaxis and by what means.

Treatment

Anticoagulation   Full anticoagulation of a postoperative patient has the risk of haematoma formation in relation to the wound. Full anticoagulation in the elderly has the risk of a cerebro-vascular accident due to an intracranial bleed. In the elderly, with a clot in the calf veins, the risk of a pulmonary embolism is small. Consequently, not all surgeons treat all deep vein thromboses. You should check with the surgeon before commencing full anticoagulation in the elderly, as once started it is difficult to stop.

Other relative contra-indications to anticoagulation are a history of haematemesis, peptic ulceration, haematuria, hypertension and women in their first trimester or last 4 weeks of pregnancy.

Full anticoagulation with heparin gives considerable pain relief and the swelling and redness usually settle within 48 hours.

If the diagnosis of a deep vein thrombosis is seriously being considered in a patient who would be treated should they have a thrombosis, but a venogram cannot be obtained until the next day (or after the weekend), treatment should be started immediately. If the venogram is normal the treatment can be discontinued.

Heparin   If the thrombosis is to be treated, start a continuous intravenous infusion of heparin in a dose of 100–150 i.u. per kg body weight every 6 hours. For most adults, a suitable regime would be 10 000 units intravenously as a loading dose followed by an infusion giving 30–40 000 units per day. Measure the KCCT after 4–6 hours, and then daily, aiming to keep it to two to three times the normal level.

Warfarin

Surgeons differ as to when they think that warfarin should be started. Some start it with the heparin, since it will take some days for the dose to stabilize. Some prefer to delay starting the warfarin for 5 days to allow the heparin to have full therapeutic effect. Warfarin takes 24–48 hours to have a measurable effect. Patients vary in their sensitivity to warfarin and the elderly or those with a low body weight can be especially sensitive. Many drugs and conditions affect the activity of warfarin and you must be aware of possible interactions.

A therapeutic regime is to give a loading dose of 10 mg for two nights and then measure the prothrombin time ratio (patient's : standardized). The aim is to have a ratio between two and three. In many hospitals the haematologists will monitor the therapy, and even if they do not, they will be happy to advise on dosages. It is best to prescribe the warfarin to be given at 6 p.m. so that the results of the morning prothrombin ratio are available.

Upper Limb

10   Dislocation of the acromio-clavicular joint

The condition

Injury to the acromio-clavicular joint is classified as:

Grade 1   A sprain
Grade 2   A subluxation
Grade 3   A complete dislocation

Making the diagnosis

The patient

The patient is usually an athletic male who has fallen directly onto the point of the shoulder.

On examination

The patient is tender over the acromio-clavicular joint. If it is a grade 3 injury, the outer end of the clavicle may be quite prominent.

Radiographs

Order an AP view of the shoulder. A patient with a pure ligamentous sprain has a normal radiograph. A completely dislocated joint should be easily seen on an AP view of the shoulder. If there is any doubt as to the presence of a subluxation or dislocation, order weight bearing films of both the injured and the uninjured shoulder for comparison. These radiographs are taken with the patient holding a weight in each hand and show a subluxation or dislocation more clearly.

Treatment

A broad arm sling and early mobilization is all that is necessary for grade 1 and grade 2 injuries. Open reduction and internal fixation is indicated for complete dislocation in the active young adult.

Indications for surgery

Grade 3 injury, i.e. dislocation, in a young active patient (e.g. labourer or keen rugby player).

Operation: repair of a dislocation of the acromio-clavicular joint

There are several methods of operative treatment of dislocation of the acromio-clavicular joint. The joint itself, as well as the coraco-clavicular ligament, have to be exposed. The incision can either be anterior over the delto-pectoral groove, or lateral. The joint is reduced and then held, either by a screw passing through the clavicle into the coracoid process (Bosworth screw), or by threaded pins which are passed through the acromion into the clavicle. The ligaments and the capsule also have to be repaired. The fixation, whether screw or pins, has to be removed after 6 weeks. The aim is to keep the dislocation reduced whilst the soft tissues heal.

Codes

GA/LA	GA . . . .
Blood	0 . . . .
Antibiotics	Yes . . . .
Time	1 hour . . . .
Drains	0 . . . .
Plaster	0 . . . .
Postoperative radiograph .	AP shoulder . . . .
Stay	24 hours . . . .
Follow up	1 week . . . .
Off work	2–6 weeks depending on occupation . . . .

Operative requirements
Standard AO set, with a 4.5 mm lag screw or threaded pins.

Postoperative care
Management
The arm is rested in a broad arm sling for 1 week. Then gentle shoulder and elbow exercises are started, avoiding full elevation until the internal fixation is removed.
Readmit after 6 weeks for removal of the screw/pins as a day-case under GA.

Complications
Injury to the brachial plexus.
Redislocation following removal of the screw.
Breakage of the pins or screws.

11   Dislocation of the shoulder

The condition

The most common direction for dislocation of the head of the humerus is anterior, but it may dislocate posteriorly.

Making the diagnosis

The patient

The patient is typically a young adult but not necessarily so.

The history

The first dislocation of a shoulder requires considerable force and usually follows a fall. The patient has considerable pain around the shoulder and may well suggest the diagnosis on arrival in casualty.

On examination

Look at both of the patient's shoulders. The normal contour of the dislocated shoulder is lost when compared to the uninjured one.

Test the function of the axillary nerve. Sensation is easy, i.e. sensation over the lateral part of the shoulder. Motor function is difficult to test with the shoulder dislocated. Ask the patient to gently abduct the shoulder whilst you palpate the deltoid muscle. If you feel any contraction within the deltoid, the motor supply is intact. Do not omit to also test the integrity of the median, ulnar and radial nerves.

Radiographs

An AP view of the shoulder will show the humeral head to be in an abnormal position. In an anterior dislocation, it lies inferior to the coracoid. In a posterior dislocation, the head may look as if it is in the correct place, except that its orientation makes the head look like a light bulb. Always ask for a second view. The easiest to interpret is an axillary view.

Common associated injuries

The axillary nerve may be injured when the shoulder dislocates or when it is reduced.

Indications for surgery

Treatment

Acute dislocations of the shoulder need to be reduced. The sooner this is done the easier it is to do.

Operation: reduction of dislocated shoulder

The shoulder can be reduced by a variety of techniques. Kocher's manoeuvre is most commonly used. If the shoulder cannot be reduced under intravenous sedation, it is safer to give the patient a general anaesthetic, which provides complete relaxation.

Codes

GA/LA	IV sedation or GA
Blood	0
Antibiotics	0
Time	10 minutes
Drains	0
Plaster	0
Postoperative radiograph	AP shoulder
Stay	Day case
Follow up	3 weeks
Off work	3 weeks

Management

Postoperative care

Recheck the function of the axillary nerve.

Always obtain postreduction radiographs.

Rest the arm in a sling for 3 weeks before starting gentle active exercises, avoiding external rotation combined with abduction for a further 3 weeks.

Complications

Axillary nerve injury.

Humeral fracture during reduction.

Recurrent dislocation.

Recurrent dislocation of the shoulder

The condition
If dislocation of the shoulder tears the glenoid labrum from its attachment, recurrence is very likely with little or no trauma.

Making the diagnosis

The patient

The patient is typically a young adult male.

The history

There should be documentation of a true dislocation of the shoulder, confirmed radiologically and having required a doctor to reduce the shoulder. The importance of this evidence is to confirm that there was indeed a dislocation as opposed to a feeling of the 'shoulder coming out of joint' that may be only subluxation. The radiographs will also show if the dislocation was anterior or posterior.

On examination

Stand behind the seated patient. To examine the right shoulder, place your left hand on the patient's right shoulder with your middle finger on the coracoid process, the index on the front of the humeral head and your thumb behind the humeral head. Lift the arm into abduction with external rotation. This will produce apprehension in the patient and the humeral head will be felt to come forwards if there is true instability.

Document the integrity of the axillary nerve, i.e. intact sensation over the deltoid muscle and motor function of the deltoid, as the nerve can be damaged with dislocation.

Radiographs

Order AP and axillary views of the shoulder. A dent in the posterior part of the humeral head is a sign of recurrent anterior dislocation.

Treatment

Indications for surgery

Multiple dislocations of the shoulder that interfere with the patient's daily activities. The patient must be made aware that there will be some loss of external rotation and that there will be a sizeable scar following surgery.

Operation: stabilization of the shoulder for recurrent dislocation

The shoulder is exposed through an anterior bra-strap incision.

1 In the Putti–Platt operation, the subscapularis tendon and anterior capsule that run across the front of the shoulder are divided. They are tightened by being sutured back together in a double-breasted fashion.

2 In the Bankart procedure, an attempt is made to correct the underlying lesion by reattaching the detached glenoid labrum to the glenoid.

3 In the Bristow procedure, the coracoid process is detached and reattached to the front of the glenoid to form a bony block to further anterior dislocation.

Codes

GA/LA	GA . . . .
Blood	Group and save . . . .
Antibiotics	Optional . . . .
Time	1½ hours . . . .
Drains	Occasionally . . . .
Plaster	0 . . . .
Postoperative radiograph .	0 . . . .
Stay	3 days . . . .
Follow up	2 weeks . . . .
Off work	6 weeks . . . .

Postoperative care

Management

Check the integrity of the musculo-cutaneous nerve by asking the patient to contract their biceps.

Elbow, wrist and hand exercises are started immediately.

The arm is held in a sling that prevents any external rotation for 6 weeks, and then the patient is allowed to self-mobilize.

Complications   Neuro-vascular injury, especially to the musculo-cutaneous nerve.
Recurrent dislocation (approximately 5%).

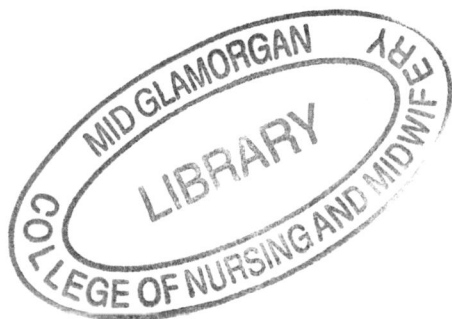

13   Tear of the rotator cuff of the shoulder

The condition
The rotator cuff comprises the tendons of supraspinatus, infraspinatus and teres minor. Tears occur in a cuff that is degenerate, usually following an acute event such as a fall.

Making the diagnosis

The patient
The patient is usually middle aged.

The history
The patient injures the shoulder whilst protecting him/herself in a fall. If the patient feels that it is only a sprain, they may not seek a medical opinion until months later after the symptoms have failed to settle. The typical picture is a patient who cannot actively abduct beyond 20–30 degrees. They complain of not being able to reach up for things on a shelf or to brush their hair.

On examination
Whilst active abduction is markedly reduced, you should be able to passively abduct the arm past 90 degrees. At this point the patient may be able to keep the arm raised by use of the deltoid.

Radiographs
Order an AP view of the shoulder. Avulsion of the greater tuberosity of the humeral head is pathognomonic of a torn rotator cuff. This is seen with the minority of torn cuffs.

In patients who are seen after the acute event, a plain AP radiograph may show a diminished space between the humeral head and the acromion. This suggests that the cuff is torn and no longer separates the humeral head from the acromion. If in doubt, obtain a view of the normal side for comparison.

The definitive investigation is the double contrast arthrogram. If there is a tear, the contrast is seen to pass out of the shoulder joint into the subacromial bursa.

**Indications for
surgery**

Treatment

A complete tear of the rotator cuff demonstrated on the arthrogram, in a patient who has pain and weakness.

Operation: repair of the torn rotator cuff of the shoulder

Some surgeons approach the shoulder through a vertical but lateral incision that splits the acromion. Others prefer the less cosmetic bra-strap incision that runs over the delto-pectoral groove. The cuff is mobilized and repaired. This can be difficult in a cuff that is very degenerate.

Codes

GA/LA	GA
Blood	Group and save
Antibiotics	Yes
Time	1 hour
Drains	0
Plaster	0
Postoperative radiograph	0
Stay	3–5 days
Follow up	3 weeks
Off work	8 weeks

**Operative
requirements**

The patient should be in the deck-chair position with a sand-bag under the shoulder that is being operated upon.

Management

Postoperative care

The arm should be rested in a sling that includes a circumferential body strap to prevent external rotation of the arm. When the pain has subsided, gentle pendulum exercises are begun. After 3 weeks active assisted exercises are begun.

Complications

Neuro-vascular damage.
Wound infection.
Re-rupture.
Stiffness.

14

Arthritis of the shoulder

The condition

Severe arthritis of the shoulder is common in patients with rheumatoid arthritis. Primary osteoarthritis of the shoulder is uncommon, but secondary osteoarthritis can follow trauma to the shoulder.

Making the diagnosis

The patient

The patient usually has polyarticular rheumatoid arthritis involving other upper limb joints.

The history

The most significant symptom is pain. This is usually accompanied by stiffness. Daily activities such as brushing the hair or getting the hand to the mouth may be impossible. You should also ask whether the patient can perform 'personal hygiene' after going to the toilet.

On examination

Examine the active range of movement of the shoulder. Fix the scapula with one hand whilst assisting with the range of movements to distinguish between scapulo-thoracic and gleno-humeral movement.

Examine the upper limbs in total, as other more severely affected joints may require surgery first.

Radiographs

AP and axillary views of the shoulder.

Preoperative management

Preparation for surgery

If the patient has rheumatoid arthritis, examine the range of neck and temporo-mandibular movements. Ensure that there are a recent set of cervical spine radiographs to exclude cervical instability.

Treatment

Indications for surgery

Severe pain in the shoulder that is unrelieved by conservative measures, i.e. physiotherapy and intra-articular steroid injections.

Operation: total shoulder replacement

The shoulder is accessible through an anterior bra-strap incision after division of the subscapularis tendon and the anterior capsule. The articular surface of the humeral head is removed, and a metal humeral pros-thesis, similar to the femoral component of a total hip replacement, is inserted down the shaft of the humerus. The glenoid component is either totally plastic or metal backed, depending on the design of the prosthesis. The components can be inserted with or without cement.

Codes

GA/LA	GA
Blood	Group and save
Antibiotics	Yes
Time	1½ hours
Drains	Yes
Plaster	0
Postoperative radiograph	AP and lateral shoulder
Stay	3 weeks
Follow up	6 weeks
Off work	3 months

Operative requirements

Arrange the patient in the astronaut/deck-chair posi-tion, with a sand-bag under the shoulder to be operated upon.

Postoperative care

Management

Check the integrity of the median, radial and ulnar nerves. The upper limb is rested in a sling for 5 days. Gentle mobilization is then commenced. The patient can be discharged home when they can touch their nose and when they can hold a cup of tea.

Complications

Nerve injury.
Infection.
Dislocation.
Loosening.

15

Fractured shaft of humerus

The patient

Making the diagnosis
The fracture may be an isolated low velocity injury or may be part of multiple trauma.

The history
The patient may have suffered a direct blow on the upper arm, may have fallen onto the arm or have been in a road traffic accident.

On examination
The diagnosis of the fracture itself is usually obvious.
Examine the contour of the shoulder to exclude an associated dislocation.
Examine the function of the radial nerve; i.e. sensation over the dorsum of the hand, plus active wrist dorsiflexion and metacarpophalangeal joint extension.

Radiographs
Ensure that the whole humerus has been X-rayed. Both the shoulder and the elbow must be included.

Common associated injuries

Preoperative management
Radial nerve neurapraxia or division.

Preparation for surgery
Depending on the instability of the fracture and the time until surgery, immobilize the arm in either a U-slab or just a collar and cuff.

Treatment
The majority of isolated humeral shaft fractures can be managed as an out-patient in a collar and cuff.

Indications for surgery
Patient with multiple injuries.
Unacceptable position of fracture after a trial of conservative therapy in a collar and cuff or plaster immobilization.
Delayed/non-union.
If the radial nerve ceases to function either immediately following the fracture, or after manipulation of the

fracture, it must be explored and repaired if necessary. The fracture has to be stabilized in order to allow the nerve to be repaired.

Operation: internal fixation of fractured shaft of humerus

The precise method of fixation depends on the fracture and the surgeon. The choice is either open plating of the fracture or closed reduction and insertion of an intramedullary nail. The nail can either be inserted from above, through the non-articular part of the humeral head, or from below, through the olecranon fossa.

Codes

GA/LA	GA
Blood	2 units
Antibiotics	Yes
Time	1½ hours
Drains	Yes
Plaster	0
Postoperative radiograph	AP and lateral humerus
Stay	3–4 days
Follow up	2 weeks
Off work	8 weeks

Operative requirements

If a closed procedure (insertion of an intramedullary nail) is to be performed, then the image intensifier and a radiographer are required.

Postoperative care

Management

Check the integrity of the radial nerve in recovery.

Encourage mobilization of the whole limb if the fixation is stable and a nerve repair has not been performed. Otherwise immobilize the upper limb with an above-elbow cast for 3–6 weeks.

Complications

Injury to the radial nerve.

Infection.

Inadequate fixation.

Non-union.

16

Supracondylar fracture of the humerus

The condition
A fracture of the distal humerus that may, or may not, extend into the elbow joint.

The patient

Making the diagnosis
This fracture is common in children who fall onto the outstretched arm. The fracture is often minimally displaced and is not usually comminuted. By contrast, this fracture is uncommon in adults, when it occurs as a result of a high energy injury such as a fall from a height or a motorcycle accident.

On examination
The elbow may be grossly swollen. Examine and document the presence of the radial pulse and the intact function of the radial, median and ulnar nerves.

Radiographs
Order AP and lateral views of the whole humerus. It is essential in children and often helpful in adults to ask for radiographs of the uninjured elbow for comparison.

Common associated injuries

Preoperative management
Entrapment or division of the brachial artery.

Preparation for surgery
Place the arm in an above-elbow back-slab with the arm in whatever position is most confortable, until the patient goes to theatre. Make sure that the radial pulse is still present after the back-slab has been applied.

Treatment
In a child with an undisplaced crack, or a fracture that is angulated less than 20 degrees on the lateral view, an above-elbow back-slab with a collar and cuff is sufficient. This is kept on for 3 weeks and then the arm is mobilized.

A fracture that is only angulated on the lateral view

of the elbow can usually be manipulated into a satisfactory position.

If a displaced fracture can be reduced, but once reduced seems unstable, the position can be held with K-wires. These are left protruding through the skin for ease of removal.

If the fracture cannot be reduced closed, an open reduction may be necessary, and this must be included on the consent.

If the fracture cannot be reduced and the arm is very swollen, the arm should be put on traction using either skin traction or a traction screw inserted into the coranoid process of the ulna.

Indications for surgery

Displaced fracture.

Comminuted fracture that can be reconstructed.

Operation: manipulation under anaesthesia of supracondylar fracture of the humerus in a child

The arm is manipulated and the position is checked with the image intensifier. The arm should be immobilized in a collar and cuff with the elbow flexed. Since excessive flexion may occlude the brachial artery, the degree of elbow flexion is a compromise between stability and vascularity.

Codes

GA/LA	GA
Blood	0
Antibiotics	0
Time	½ hour
Drains	0
Plaster	Above elbow
Postoperative radiograph	AP and lateral elbow
Stay	2 nights
Follow up	1 week, X-ray on arrival
Off school	2 weeks

Operative requirements

Image intensifier and radiographer.

Management

Postoperative care

The major risk following manipulation of this fracture is the development of a compartment syndrome. Carefully check the movement of the fingers. Loss of full extension of the fingers due to pain is the first sign of a compartment syndrome. If the child has increasing pain, do not just give stronger analgesics, but carefully assess the child and if at all concerned, call a more senior person.

Complications

Compartment syndrome.
Loss of position.
Abnormal growth leading to a gun-stock deformity.

Operation: open reduction and K-wiring of supracondylar fracture of the humerus in a child

The fracture is reduced through a lateral incision plus/minus a medial incision. Once reduced, two K-wires are inserted. The reduction and the position of the wires is checked with the image intensifier.

Codes

GA/LA	GA . . . .
Blood	Group and save . . . .
Antibiotics	Yes . . . .
Time	1 hour . . . .
Drains	0 . . . .
Plaster	Above-elbow back-slab . .
Postoperative radiograph . .	AP and lateral elbow . . . .
Stay	3 days . . . .
Follow up	1 week . . . .
Off school	2 weeks . . . .

Operative requirements

K-wires and Jacob's chuck.

Management

Postoperative care

The major risk following open reduction of this fracture is the development of a compartment syndrome. Care-

fully check the sensation and movement of the fingers.
If the child has increasing pain, do not just give stronger
analgesics, but carefully assess the child and if at all
concerned, call a more senior person.

Complications   Compartment syndrome.
Loss of position.
Abnormal growth leading to a gun-stock deformity.

Operation: insertion of olecranon skeletal traction screw for supracondylar fracture of the humerus

A small incision is made over the ulna opposite the
coranoid process. A screw is inserted perpendicular to
the long axis of the ulna, to which traction is attached.

Codes

GA/LA................	GA	
Blood	0	
Antibiotics	0	
Time.................	½ hour	
Drains................	0	
Stay..................	2 weeks	
Postoperative radiograph ..	AP and lateral elbow in traction	
Follow up	1 week, X-ray on arrival ..	

Operative   Small fragment AO malleolar screw.
requirements   Set up the traction on the bed prior to the procedure
so that the patient can be placed on traction whilst
anaesthetized.

Postoperative care
Management   *Beware compartment syndrome* — if patient has increasing
pain, and the fingers cannot be passively extended,
call a senior person. Do not just give stronger
analgesics.
Arrange longitudinal traction on the ulna with 1.5–
2.5 kg (3–5 lb), plus skin traction on forearm to

maintain the elbow at approximately 45 degrees with
0.5–1 kg (1–2 lb).

Traction is maintained for 2 weeks and then the patient
is discharged home in an above-elbow plaster in
which they remain for 1 further week.

Complications   Compartment syndrome.

Loss of position.

Abnormal growth; a varus deformity is the commonest
and cosmetically most unacceptable deformity.

17   Tennis elbow

The condition
This condition is due to repetitive strain.

Making the diagnosis

The history   Tennis elbow is characterized by pain that is maximal over the lateral epicondyle of the elbow. There will have been a gradual onset of pain that occurs with certain movements and may radiate down the whole forearm.

On examination   There is a localized area of tenderness slightly distal to the lateral epicondyle.
Stretching the extensor muscles by extending the elbow, and palmar flexing the wrist is painful. This pain is increased by getting the patient to maintain this position against resistance.

Radiographs   AP and lateral views of the elbow are necessary to exclude an alternative cause for the pain. These are usually normal.

Treatment
Conservative treatment is always the first line. Options include physiotherapy, local injection of lignocaine and steroid, and rest in a sling.

Indications for surgery   Persistent or recurrent pain that has failed to respond to conservative treatment.

Operation: release of the extensor origin for tennis elbow

A curved incision is made on the lateral side of the elbow. The origin of the extensor muscles is elevated from the bone and allowed to heal in a slightly more distal position.

Codes

GA/LA	GA . . . .
Blood	0 . . . .
Antibiotics	0 . . . .
Time	½ hour . . . .
Drains	0 . . . .
Plaster	Above elbow . . . .
Postoperative radiograph .	0 . . . .
Stay	1 night . . . .
Follow up	2 weeks . . . .
Off work	2 weeks . . . .

Operative requirements

Above-elbow tourniquet.

Management

Postoperative care

Check the integrity of the posterior interosseous nerve — can the patient actively dorsiflex the wrist?

Encourage finger mobilization.

An above-elbow plaster, with the elbow at 90 degrees, is retained for 2 weeks. The elbow is then gently mobilized.

Complications

The posterior interosseous nerve is at risk and may be bruised or even divided, leading to a wrist drop.

18   Fractured olecranon

The condition

A fracture of the olecranon usually extends into the elbow joint, and is in essence an avulsion fracture of the triceps insertion. The proximal fragment usually displaces proximally, due to the pull of the triceps.

Making the diagnosis

The history

A fall onto the point of the elbow.

On examination

There will be considerable bruising and swelling around the elbow. Test the ability of the patient to actively extend the elbow. Active extension is absent in displaced fractures.

It is important to examine and document the integrity of ulnar nerve sensation (ulnar one and a half fingers) and motor function (finger abduction).

Radiographs

AP and lateral of the elbow.

Preoperative management

Preparation for surgery

The arm must be rested, prior to surgery, in a well-padded back-slab with the elbow at 90 degrees.

Treatment

Indications for surgery

A displaced fracture.

Operation: tension band wiring of fractured olecranon

A midline posterior incision is used. The fragments are reduced and then held with two K-wires and a crossed wire loop that increases the compression on the fracture when the elbow is flexed — hence 'tension band' wiring.

Codes

GA/LA................	GA ....
Blood	0 ....
Antibiotics	Yes ....
Time................	1 hour..............
Drains................	Yes ....
Plaster................	Above elbow..........
Postoperative radiograph ...	AP and lateral elbow ...
Stay....................	3 days ....
Follow up	2 weeks..............
Off work	4 weeks.............

Operative requirements

K-wire set.

Tourniquet high on upper arm.

Some surgeons prefer to check the reduction in theatre with an on-table radiograph or with the image intensifier. If so, warn the radiographer.

Management

Postoperative care

If the fixation is solid, gentle active mobilization can begin immediately. Otherwise the arm is kept in the back-slab for 3 weeks.

Complications

Failure to achieve anatomical reduction.

Division of the ulnar nerve.

Failure of fixation.

19   Fracture of the radial head

The history

Making the diagnosis

The patient has usually fallen onto the outstretched hand and will complain of pain around the elbow.

On examination

Feel for tenderness over the radial head.

Examine the range of pronation and supination, which may be restricted by pain.

Radiographs

If a fracture is suspected, ask for AP and lateral views of the elbow as well as oblique 'radial head views'.

Investigations

Preoperative management

Aspiration of the haemarthrosis and insertion of a few millilitres of lignocaine will greatly relieve the patient's agony. In addition, this permits assessment of the range of supination and pronation whilst uninhibited by pain. If there is a full range of movement, surgery cannot improve things, whatever the fracture looks like on the radiograph.

Preparation for surgery

Rest the elbow in a well-padded back-slab prior to surgery.

Treatment

Undisplaced fractures can be rested in an above-elbow back-slab for 1 or 2 weeks, prior to beginning mobilization.

Indications for surgery

A displaced fracture with a block to rotation of the forearm when examined under local anaesthesia.

Operation: open reduction and internal fixation of a fractured radial head

The fracture is exposed through a lateral incision centred over the radial head. If possible, the fragments are reduced and then held using mini-fragment screws. The aim is to reconstruct the joint surface.

57

If the fracture is so comminuted that reconstruction is not possible, the radial head may have to be excised. The patient should be aware of this. Some surgeons like to put in an artificial replacement if the head is removed. This acts as a spacer and maintains the correct relationship between the radius and ulna.

Codes

GA/LA	GA ....
Blood	0 ....
Antibiotics	Yes ....
Time	1 hour ....
Drains	0 ....
Plaster	Above elbow ....
Postoperative radiograph .	AP and lateral elbow .....
Stay	2 days ....
Follow up.............	2 weeks ....
Off work	3 weeks ....

Operative requirements

Mini-fragment AO set.
High-arm tourniquet.

Postoperative care

Management

A plaster back-slab, that is above elbow, with the elbow at 90 degrees and extending to the metacarpophalangeal joints, is kept on for 2 weeks, prior to mobilization of the elbow.

Complications

Damage to the posterior interosseous nerve leading to a wrist drop.
Loss of fixation.
Infection.
Long-term risk of osteoarthritis.

Arthritis involving the radial head

The condition
This is commonly part of rheumatoid arthritis, but may be secondary to a previous fracture of the radial head.

Making the diagnosis

The patient The patient usually suffers from widespread rheumatoid arthritis.

The history Pain on pronation and supination, with a restricted range of movement.

On examination Examine the range of flexion and extension of the elbow, and pronation and supination of the forearm. Feel for possible crepitus with movement. If the arthritis affects the whole elbow, there may be a flexion contracture and also instability of the collateral ligaments.

Radiographs AP and lateral views of the elbow are sufficient.

Preoperative management

Investigations If the patient has rheumatoid arthritis, examine the range of neck and temporo-mandibular movements. Ensure that there are a recent set of cervical spine radiographs to exclude instability.

Treatment
The initial treatment is conservative and includes physiotherapy, splintage to restrict rotation and intra-articular steroid injection.

Indications for surgery Pain originating from the radio-humeral joint that has not responded to conservative treatment.

Operation: excision of the head of the radius

The capsule and part of the annular ligament are divided through a lateral incision centred over the radial head. The neck of the radius is divided, the head removed and the end of the radius smoothed off. Nothing is inserted into the gap created.

Codes

GA/LA................	GA ....
Blood	0 ....
Antibiotics	0 ....
Time	½ hour ....
Drains	0 ....
Plaster	Above-elbow back-slab ..
Postoperative radiograph ..	0 ....
Stay	2 days ....
Follow up	2 weeks ....
Off work	2–4 weeks ....

Operative requirements

High arm tourniquet.

Management

Postoperative care

The arm is rested in an above-elbow plaster back-slab, that extends up to the metacarpal heads with the elbow at 90 degrees, for 2 weeks. The patient then gently mobilizes the elbow.

Complications

Injury to the posterior interosseous nerve, resulting in a wrist drop.

21   Arthritis of the elbow

The condition
Severe arthritis of the elbow is common in patients with rheumatoid arthritis. Primary osteoarthritis of the elbow is rare, but degeneration may be secondary to trauma to the elbow.

Making the diagnosis

The patient
The patient usually has polyarticular arthritis involving other upper limb joints.

The history
The most significant symptom is pain. This is usually accompanied by stiffness. Daily activities such as brushing the hair or getting the hand to the mouth may be impossible. You should ask whether the patient can perform 'personal hygiene' after going to the toilet.

On examination
Examine the range of flexion and extension of the elbow, and pronation and supination of the forearm. Feel for crepitus with movement. There may be a flexion contracture and also instability of the collateral ligaments.
Carefully examine the motor and sensory function of the ulnar nerve. If the nerve is compressed it may need to be transposed.

Radiographs
AP and lateral views of the elbow are sufficient to show the considerable bony erosion that may have occurred.

Preoperative management

Investigations
If the patient has rheumatoid arthritis, examine the range of neck and temporo-mandibular movements. Ensure that there are a recent set of cervical spine radiographs to exclude instability.

Treatment

Indications for surgery
In the early stages of rheumatoid arthritis affecting the elbow, a synovectomy can give considerable pain relief and in addition delay the destruction of the joint. Once

there is severe bony destruction of the joint, that is accompanied by pain, a total elbow replacement can be performed.

Operation: total elbow replacement (Roper–Tuke)

The elbow is exposed through a posterior midline incision. The end of the humerus is prepared so as to take a metal hemicylindrical prosthesis that is cemented in place. This articulates with a plastic ulnar component that sits in the coronoid fossa and is held with a screw that passes down the shaft of the ulna.

Codes

GA/LA	GA ....
Blood	Group and save ....
Antibiotics	Yes ....
Time	1½ hours ....
Drains	Yes ....
Plaster	Above elbow ....
Postoperative radiograph .	AP and lateral elbow .....
Stay	3 weeks ....
Follow up.............	6 weeks ....
Off work	3 months ....

Operative requirements

High arm tourniquet.

Management

Postoperative care

Check that the ulnar nerve is intact by testing sensation in the ulnar one and a half fingers and the power of finger abduction.

The elbow is rested in a back-slab for 3 weeks, after which time it is gently mobilized.

Complications

Ulnar nerve dysfunction.
Instability of the elbow.
Loosening.
Infection.
Dislocation.

22   Compression of the ulnar nerve at the elbow

The condition
The ulnar nerve can be compressed as it passes through the cubital tunnel. Sensory symptoms usually precede motor symptoms.

Making the diagnosis

The history
The patient complains of numbness in the ulnar nerve distribution and of weakness in the hand. There may be a history of previous bony trauma, commonly a supracondylar fracture of the humerus which has resulted in a valgus elbow.

On examination
Examine the alignment and range of movement of the elbow.

Examine the ulnar nerve sensory and motor function of both arms; i.e. sensation in the ulnar one and a half fingers, power in the long flexor to the little finger and power of abductor digiti minimi. In severe cases there may be wasting of the first dorsal interosseous muscle or even an ulnar claw hand.

Investigations
An electromyogram will establish the site and nature of the lesion.

Radiographs
AP and lateral views of the elbow.

Treatment

Indications for surgery
Persistent symptoms of ulnar nerve dysfunction confirmed by an abnormal electromyogram.

Operation: decompression +/− transposition of the ulnar nerve

The nerve is exposed through an incision made directly over it. The commonly performed procedures are:

1 Simple decompression of the nerve in the cubital tunnel without transposition.

2 Anterior subcutaneous transposition.

3 Anterior submuscular transposition, with the nerve being placed under the flexor muscles. This submuscular anterior transposition has the longest recovery period.

Codes

GA/LA	GA . . . .
Blood	0 . . . .
Antibiotics	0 . . . .
Time	1 hour . . . .
Drains	0 . . . .
Plaster	Above elbow . . . .
Postoperative radiograph .	0 . . . .
Stay	2 days . . . .
Follow up	2 weeks . . . .
Off work	3 weeks . . . .

Operative requirements

High arm tourniquet.

Postoperative care

Management

Check the motor and sensory function of the ulnar nerve.

The arm is immobilized by an above-elbow back-slab for 2 weeks prior to gentle active mobilization.

Complications

Temporary or permanent worsening of the ulnar nerve dysfunction.

23 Olecranon bursitis

The condition
The olecranon bursa may become inflamed as a result of friction or pressure. Other uncommon causes include gout, in which the lump may be calcified, or rheumatoid arthritis.

Making the diagnosis

The history
The history is of episodes of recurrent swelling and pain. The bursa may become secondarily infected.

On examination
The bursa is over the very point of the elbow. If not presently inflamed, it may be looser and more sack like than normal, with a thickened wall.

Radiographs
A lateral radiograph of the elbow may show calcification within the bursa.

Treatment
Most episodes of inflammation can be managed conservatively with a combination of an oral non-steroidal anti-inflammatory drug, aspiration of the bursa and injection of steroid into the bursa.

Indications for surgery
Recurrent bursitis that has not responded to conservative treatment.

Operation: excision of the olecranon bursa
The bursa is completely excised through a longitudinal posterior incision.

Codes

GA/LA	GA . . . .
Blood	0 . . . .
Antibiotics	Optional . . . .
Time	30 minutes . . . .
Drains	Yes . . . .

Plaster	0 . . . .
Postoperative radiograph .	0 . . . .
Stay	2 days . . . .
Follow up	2 weeks . . . .
Off work	3 weeks . . . .

Operative
requirements

Tourniquet.

Management

Postoperative care

The dressings are reduced and the drain is removed after 24 hours. Immediate mobilization of the elbow is encouraged, but the elbow can be rested in a sling between times.

Complications

Wound infection.
Wound haematoma.
Injury to the ulnar nerve.

24   Fracture of the shafts of the radius and ulna

The condition
When both bones of the forearm are fractured, they may be either displaced or undisplaced. If a single bone is broken and is displaced, there must be another discontinuity in the rectangle formed by the radius, the ulna, and the proximal and distal radio-ulnar joints. A Monteggia fracture is the combination of a proximal ulnar fracture with dislocation of the radial head at the elbow. A Galeazzi fracture is a fracture of the distal radius with dislocation of the distal ulna.

Making the diagnosis

The patient This fracture can occur in a patient of any age.

On examination The diagnosis is usually clinically obvious:
Examine the neuro-vascular integrity of the hand. Restriction in extension of the fingers or diminished sensation may be indicative of a compartment syndrome and urgent decompression may be necessary.
Note the presence and location of any grazes or fracture blisters, as these may prevent immediate open reduction.

Radiographs Obtain AP and lateral views of the whole forearm with the wrist and elbow included. Look for dislocation of the radial head at the elbow or the ulna at the wrist.

Preoperative management

Common associated injuries Compartment syndrome.
Injury to the nerves or vessels of the forearm.

Preparation for surgery Rest and immobilize the arm in a well-padded above-elbow back-slab.

Treatment

Indications for surgery In children, angulation on the lateral radiograph may be acceptable. The younger the patient, the greater the potential for remodelling with growth and therefore the greater the angulation which can be accepted. However, if the arm looks bent, it is often best to manipulate the fracture so that the arm is straight. This is because parents often do not believe that it will grow straight.

Deformity that is varus or valgus, or rotational will not remodel with growth and therefore must be corrected.

In adults, only completely undisplaced fractures of both bones are treated conservatively in a plaster. All others are reduced and internally fixed.

Operation: manipulation under anaesthesia of fractured radius and ulna in a child

The fracture is manipulated under a general anaesthetic and the position checked with the image intensifier. The limb is then immobilized in a well-padded above-elbow back-slab, or a full plaster that is split.

Codes

GA/LA	GA . . . .
Blood	0 . . . .
Antibiotics	0 . . . .
Time	½ hour . . . .
Drains	0 . . . .
Plaster	Above elbow . . . .
Postoperative radiograph . .	AP and lateral radius and ulna . . . .
Stay	1 night . . . .
Follow up	1 week, X-ray on arrival . . .
Off school	1 week . . . .

Operative requirements

Image intensifier and radiographer.

Postoperative care

Management   Elevate the arm on pillows. Instruct the nurses on careful monitoring of the neuro-vascular status of the hand. Beware compartment syndrome! An immobilized, reduced fracture should not be very painful. If there is increasing pain, do not just increase the analgesics, but go and see the patient. If concerned call the surgeon.

Complications

Compartment syndrome.
Loss of position.
Malunion.
Restricted pronation or supination due to persistent rotational malunion.

Operation: open reduction and internal fixation of the radius and ulna in an adult

The ulna is exposed through an incision over the subcutaneous border of the bone. The radius is approached through either an anterior or a lateral incision. The vital structures such as the radial artery and radial nerve have to be seen and protected as part of the anterior exposure of the radius. The fractures are reduced and then held using plates and screws.

Codes

GA/LA...............	GA ....
Blood	0 ....
Antibiotics	Yes ....
Time.................	1½ hours ....
Drains................	Yes ....
Plaster................	0 ....
Postoperative radiograph ..	AP and lateral radius and ulna ....
Stay..................	3 days ....
Follow up	2 weeks ....
Off work	4 weeks ....

Operative requirements

Small fragment AO set.
High arm tourniquet.

Postoperative care

Management

Elevate the arm on two pillows.
Carefully monitor the neuro-vascular function in the hand.

Beware compartment syndrome.

Encourage immediate mobilization of the hand and elbow.

Complications   Compartment syndrome.

Neurapraxia or division of the radial, ulnar or median nerve.

Infection.

Non-union.

Late fracture of the forearm at the plate/non-plate junction.

Removal of internal fixation of the forearm

The condition

Following union of a fracture that has been fixed with a plate, there is an increased risk of fracture of the bone at the point where the plate ends. This is because the plate acts as a stress riser. In other words, due to the plate's rigidity, the force of the fall is concentrated at one point. Fixation of these fractures is difficult. Therefore, in the young, it is best to remove the plates after union of the fracture. However, removal of plates is associated with a greater risk of nerve injury than the original operation. This is because scar tissue makes identification of vital structures difficult.

Treatment

Indications for surgery

A healed forearm fracture, at least 18 months following internal fixation, in a patient less than 40 years.

Operation: removal of plates from radius and ulna

The plates are exposed and removed through the original incisions.

Codes

GA/LA................	GA.................
Blood	0....................
Antibiotics	0....................
Time	45 minutes...........
Drains	Yes.................
Plaster................	0....................
Postoperative radiograph ..	AP and lateral forearm ..
Stay...................	2 days...............
Follow up	10 days..............
Off work..............	3 weeks ....

Operative requirements

Tourniquet.
Screwdriver of the appropriate size and type. In general, this will be the screwdriver for the AO small fragment screws.

Management

Postoperative care

The arm does not need immobilization.

The patient must be aware that following the removal of the plates, the bones can fracture with less force than is required to break a normal bone. This is because the bone that was under the plates has been shielded from stress and is thus weaker than normal. It takes 3–6 months for the bones to regain normal strength. The patient can use the arm for normal activities immediately postoperatively, but should do no sport for 3 months and avoid extreme activities for 6 months.

Complications

The incidence of complications following removal of plates is much higher than following their insertion:

Nerve injury.

Wound infection.

Unsightly scar.

Refracture.

26 Fracture/separation of the epiphysis of the distal radius

The condition
This is the equivalent in children of a Colles' fracture in an adult.

Making the diagnosis

The patient
A child between 8 years old and their teens.

The history
The history will be of a fall onto the outstretched hand. The child will complain of a painful wrist.

On examination
The wrist is swollen, painful and may be deformed. Gently examine the whole forearm and elbow to exclude a more proximal injury.

Radiographs
Obtain AP and lateral views of the wrist. If only one bone is fractured at the wrist, there may be a fracture more proximally. Beware missing a Galeazzi combination of a fractured radius with dislocation of the distal radio-ulnar joint. If in doubt X-ray the whole forearm and also the uninjured side for comparison.

Preoperative management

Preparation for surgery
Rest the wrist in a well-padded below-elbow back-slab.

Treatment
The younger the child, the greater the potential for remodelling with growth. Therefore if the displacement is minimal, the added trauma of a manipulation may not be necessary and may in fact further injure the growth plate.

Indications for surgery
A fracture that is significantly displaced.

73

Operation: manipulation under anaesthesia of a fractured distal radius in a child

The wrist is gently manipulated. Flexion of the fracture is usually the only manoeuvre necessary. The reduction is checked with the image intensifier and a plaster cast is applied which is immediately split.

Codes

GA/LA	GA . . . .
Blood	0 . . . .
Antibiotics	0 . . . .
Time	½ hour . . . .
Drains	0 . . . .
Plaster	Above elbow . . . .
Postoperative radiograph . .	AP and lateral wrist . . . . .
Stay	1 night . . . .
Follow up	1 week, X-ray on arrival . . .
Off school	1 week . . . .

Operative requirements

Image intensifier and radiographer.

Management

Postoperative care

Elevate the arm and encourage early finger movement.

Carefully monitor the neuro-vascular status of the hand. Beware compartment syndrome!

The length of time that the cast is kept on depends on the age of the child. In young children, 3 weeks is adequate. In teenagers, 6 weeks is necessary.

Complications

Compartment syndrome.

Loss of position.

Colles' fracture

The condition
A fracture of the distal radius that is 2.5 cm (1 in.) from the wrist joint, with the distal fragment being dorsally tilted, impacted, and often radially displaced.

Making the diagnosis

The patient Typically, a postmenopausal woman.

The history A fall onto an outstretched hand resulting in a painful wrist.

On examination The wrist is usually swollen. If the fracture is grossly displaced, there will be a 'dinner fork' deformity. Examine the neuro-vascular status of the hand as an acute carpal tunnel syndrome can occur, with resultant paraesthesia in the radial three and a half fingers.

Radiographs Order AP and lateral radiographs of the wrist. When looking at the lateral view:
Ensure that the orientation is correct, i.e. with the forearm horizontal and the thumb pointing down. In this position, the distal fragment will be tipped up and back if it is a Colles' fracture. If it is tipped down, you are looking at a Smith's fracture.
Ensure that the crescentic outline of the lunate is in line with the radius and in line with capitate. If it is not, it may be dislocated downwards and pressing on the median nerve!

Preoperative management

Common associated injuries Other fractures associated with osteoporosis, in particular the neck of the femur.

Preparation for surgery Rest the wrist in a back-slab.

Treatment

If the fracture is undisplaced, the wrist is simply immobilized in a below-elbow cast.

If the fracture is displaced, it may need to be reduced. The amount of displacement that is acceptable increases with the age of the patient. In a 40 year old, no displacement is acceptable. In a 90 year old, considerable displacement is accepted.

In a fracture that is not comminuted, manipulation and application of a cast is usually sufficient.

If the fracture has a lot of dorsal comminution, so that it is likely to redisplace, the reduction can be held with percutaneous K-wires.

If the whole fracture is comminuted, the radius can be held out to length using an external fixator.

Indications for surgery

A fracture that is significantly displaced.

A fracture previously manipulated, which has lost its position.

Operation: manipulation under anaesthesia of Colles' fracture +/− application of external fixator or insertion of K-wires

When a Colles' fracture is manipulated, the aim is to:

1 Restore the radius to its proper length in relation to the ulna on the AP view of the wrist.

2 Restore the angle of the articular surface of the radius to 15 degrees of palmar flexion.

If an external fixator has to be used to hold the reduction, two pins are inserted into the second metacarpal and two into the radius, proximal to the fracture.

Codes

GA/LA . . . .   GA or regional block . . .
Blood . . . .   0 . . . .
Antibiotics . . . .   0 . . . .
Time . . . .   ½ hour . . . .
Drains . . . .   0 . . . .
Plaster . . . .   Below elbow . . . .

Postoperative radiograph . . .   AP and lateral wrist . . . .
Stay . . . .   24 hours . . . .
Follow up . . . .   1 week, X-ray on arrival
Off work . . . .   2–6 weeks depending on
                                              occupation . . . .

**Operative
requirements**

Plain films or image intensifier.

Management

Postoperative care

Elevate the hand and encourage mobilization of the fingers, elbow and shoulder. A sling, if used, should be discarded after 24 hours.

If the wrist is in a cast, the fracture may redisplace up to 2 weeks following reduction. Therefore, the patient must be seen in the fracture clinic and the position checked with a radiograph after 1 and after 2 weeks. The wrist is kept in a cast for 3–6 weeks.

If the fracture has been held with K-wires or an external fixator, these are removed after 4 weeks and the wrist is immobilized in a plaster cast for a further 2 weeks.

Complications

Loss of position. This can occur up to 2 weeks after manipulation of the fracture.

Carpal tunnel syndrome.

The condition

A fracture of the distal radius that is 2.5 cm (1 in.) from the wrist joint, with the distal fragment being tilted towards the palm.

Making the diagnosis

The patient

Typically a postmenopausal woman.

The history

A fall onto the back of the hand.

On examination

The wrist is deformed. Examine the neuro-vascular status of the hand as an acute carpal tunnel syndrome is not uncommon, with resultant paraesthesia in the radial three and a half fingers.

Radiographs

Request AP and lateral radiographs of the wrist. When looking at the lateral view, ensure that the orientation is correct, i.e. with the thumb pointing down. In this position the distal fragment will be tipped down. If it is tipped up, it is a Colles' fracture.

Preoperative management

Common associated injuries

Other fractures associated with osteoporosis, in particular a fracture of the neck of the femur.

Preparation for surgery

Rest the wrist in a back-slab.

Treatment

Any fracture that is displaced needs to be reduced. Initially a closed manipulation can be performed. However, loss of position is common and the fracture then requires open reduction and internal fixation.

Indications for surgery

Open reduction and internal fixation is required if the fracture cannot be manipulated into a satisfactory position or if a good reduction has been lost.

Operation: open reduction and internal fixation of Smith's fracture

The fracture is exposed through a longitudinal incision on the front of the wrist. The fracture is reduced and then the distal fragment is held in position with a 'T' plate that acts as a buttress. The plate is only screwed to the proximal fragment, since the distal fragment is usually too porotic to hold screws.

Codes

GA/LA...............	GA ....
Blood	0 ....
Antibiotics	Yes ....
Time..................	1 hour ....
Drains................	0 ....
Plaster................	Below elbow, 6 weeks ..
Postoperative radiograph ...	AP and lateral wrist ....
Stay..................	2 days ....
Follow up	2 weeks ....
Off work	2–6 weeks depending on occupation ....

Operative requirements

Small fragment AO set or Ellis 'T' plate.
Plain films or image intensifier plus radiographer.

Postoperative care

Management

Elevate the hand and encourage finger, elbow and shoulder movement.
If used, discard the sling after 24 hours.

Complications

Loss of position.
Acute carpal tunnel syndrome.

29

Carpal tunnel syndrome

The condition
The median nerve is compressed as it passes through the carpal canal at the wrist.

Making the diagnosis

The patient
The syndrome is common in postmenopausal women, in pregnancy, in rheumatoid arthritis and following a wrist fracture. However, in 50% of the patients, no predisposing cause is found.

The history
The patient complains of pain and tingling in the fingers. This may involve all the fingers, but typically affects only the radial three and a half fingers, with sparing of the little finger. The symptoms are often worse at night, with the patient waking with a numb hand which they shake 'trying to restore the circulation'. The patient may complain of an inability to pick up a fine object such as a pin.

On examination
Examine the light touch sensation in each finger, on each half of the palmar side.

Test the power of thumb abduction.

Percuss over the median nerve at the wrist to elicit Tinel's sign. This is positive if percussion over the nerve generates paraesthesia (tingling) in the fingers.

Phalen's test is the most reliable clinical test for carpal tunnel syndrome. It is performed by holding the patient's forearm vertically and allowing their wrist and hand to fall into palmar-flexion. This may reproduce the patient's symptoms after 1 or 2 minutes.

Radiographs
AP and lateral radiographs of the wrist are necessary to exclude a bony cause for the nerve compression.

Preoperative management

Investigations
The diagnosis may be confirmed with an electromyogram.

Treatment

If symptoms have commenced during pregnancy, they usually resolve after delivery. In all patients with mild symptoms, a wrist splint (Futura splint), worn at night, may be helpful.

If the electromyogram does not show slowing of conduction in the motor component of the median nerve, a local steriod injection around the nerve at the wrist may alleviate the symptoms. Surgery reliably relieves the symptoms in patients with established median nerve compression.

Indications for surgery

Carpal tunnel syndrome, preferably proven with an electromyogram.

Operation: decompression of the carpal canal

An incision is made in the palm parallel to the thenar skin crease. The transverse carpal ligament is divided under direct vision, with the incision through the ligament being on the ulnar side of the median nerve. This is to reduce the risk of injury to the motor branch to the thumb.

Codes

GA/LA	LA or GA
Blood	0
Antibiotics	0
Time	½ hour
Drains	0
Plaster	0
Postoperative radiograph	0
Stay	Day case
Follow up	2 weeks
Off work	2 weeks

Operative requirements

High arm tourniquet.

Postoperative care

Management

Elevate the arm on two pillows.

Check the integrity of thumb abduction before the
patient is discharged.

Complications   Division of the motor nerve to the thumb.

Division of the palmar cutaneous nerve.

A feeling of weakness of grip that takes several months
to settle.

Recurrence of median nerve compression.

Wrist ganglion

The condition

A ganglion is a cyst containing viscous fluid, that is usually in continuity with the wrist joint. The lump may alter in size and although not in itself tender, may be associated with some pain around the wrist.

Making the diagnosis

The patient   Usually a young adult.

The history   The ganglion is normally on the dorsum of the wrist. It may vary in size over a period of weeks. There may be some aching on use of the wrist. Always ask if there has been any previous trauma to the wrist.

On examination   The lump is firm and not fixed to the skin but to the underlying structures. It is usually on the dorsum of the wrist but may be on the palmar aspect.

Radiographs   Always obtain AP and lateral radiographs of the wrist to exclude bony pathology and to see if there are any degenerative changes in the wrist or carpal joints.

Treatment

The ganglion can be aspirated and then injected with steroid. This is done in the clinic and has a 30% cure rate.

Indications for surgery   A persistent lump that the patient would like to have removed.

Contra-indications to surgery   A patient who is unwilling to exchange a lump for a scar. Therefore always ensure that the patient is aware that they will have a scar that will be at least as long as the diameter of the lump and that the operation site will be quite painful for some time.

Operation: excision of wrist ganglion

The ganglion is freed from the surrounding tissue and followed down to its base. Ideally this is done without bursting the ganglion, which is then excised.

Codes

GA/LA	LA ....
Blood	0 ....
Antibiotics	0 ....
Time	½ hour...............
Drains	0 ....
Plaster	0 ....
Postoperative radiograph .	0 ....
Stay	Day case ....
Follow up.............	10 days...............
Off work	10 days...............

Operative requirements

Tourniquet.

Postoperative care

Management

Elevate the hand for the first day postoperatively.

Complications

There is a real risk of recurrence after excision that may be as great as 30%.

Alternatively, a new ganglion may develop close to the site of the previous one.

Ganglions on the dorsum of the wrist have minimal additional complications.

Ganglions on the palmar aspect have a risk of adjacent vital structures being damaged when the ganglion is excised. Also, the preoperative diagnosis may have been incorrect and the mass may, for example, be a tumour of the median nerve, which should not be excised by the inexperienced.

31   Fractured scaphoid

The condition

The scaphoid is the most frequently fractured carpal bone. It is notable for the difficulty that can occur in diagnosing the fracture and for the incidence in delayed and non-union.

Making the diagnosis

The patient

Scaphoid fractures are rare in the skeletally immature (prior to closure of the epiphyses) and unusual after middle age.

The history

The patient usually recalls falling onto their outstretched hand. He will complain of a painful wrist.

On examination

The most significant signs of a scaphoid fracture are pain in the anatomical snuff box, pain over the pole of the scaphoid (felt in the base of the thenar eminence) and pain on distraction of the thumb or index finger.

Always palpate the 'normal' anatomical snuff box, as the terminal branch of the superficial nerve lies in the base and pressing on the nerve may in itself be painful. Then compare the normal with the abnormal.

Radiographs

Always request AP and lateral views of the wrist, plus 'scaphoid views'.

If clinically, the scaphoid appears to be fractured, but the radiographs are normal, it is traditional to repeat the radiographs after 10 days, when the fracture may be more easily seen.

Treatment

The majority of scaphoid fractures that are proven clinically and radiologically, are successfully treated in a below-elbow plaster cast. This extends up to the interphalangeal joint of the thumb, with the hand positioned as if holding a wine glass.

Immobilization needs to be continued until the fracture has united. This may take up to 3 months.

Indications for surgery

An established non-union of a scaphoid needs open reduction and either grafting alone or graft plus fixation with a compression screw. The exact choice depends on the nature of the fracture and the preference of the surgeon.

Operation: internal fixation and bone grafting of non-union of a scaphoid fracture with a Herbert screw

The scaphoid is exposed through an incision which crosses the wrist on the flexor aspect. Bone graft is usually taken locally from the distal radius and packed into the fracture.

The Herbert screw has a special jig to align the drill. Its main design features are the lack of a head and the differential pitch of the threads at each end, which gives compression of the fracture as the screw is tightened.

Codes

GA/LA	GA
Blood	0
Antibiotics	Yes
Time	1 hour
Drains	0
Plaster	Scaphoid below elbow
Postoperative radiograph	Scaphoid views
Stay	3 days
Follow up	2 weeks
Off work	2 weeks

Operative requirements

High arm tourniquet.
Herbert screw set.

Management

Postoperative care

Check that the screw does not come out of the proximal pole of the scaphoid into the wrist joint on the postoperative radiographs.

A scaphoid cast is usually retained for 4–6 weeks and then the patient is allowed to mobilize the wrist.

Complications   Comminution of the fracture.
Persistent non-union.

The condition
Thickening of the tendon sheath or a nodule on the flexor tendon can prevent a digit being extended from the flexed position. If the finger can be actively extended, it may extend with a sudden give, like pulling a trigger.

Making the diagnosis
The patient   Trigger thumb may occur in babies.
In adults in middle age and beyond, it is the ring and
middle fingers that are usually affected.

The history   Babies with trigger thumb are brought by their parents
with the history that the thumb will no longer
straighten.
Adults complain of pain around the base of the finger
and often state that the finger can only be straightened by using the other hand, or by using the adjacent finger.

On examination   Many patients can produce the triggering for you to see.
There may be a palpable lump on the flexor tendon just
proximal to the metacarpal head, which may be tender.

Treatment
Trigger finger in adults is often cured by an injection of
steroid around the entrance to the flexor canal. This is
done in out-patients.

Indications for   Persistent triggering despite conservative treatment.
surgery

Operation: release of trigger thumb in a baby
The first annular (A1) pulley, which forms the entrance
to the flexor sheath, is divided through a transverse or

longitudinal incision at the base of the thumb. The
tendon itself needs no treatment.

Codes

GA/LA	GA ....
Blood	0 ....
Antibiotics	0 ....
Time	20 minutes ....
Drains	0 ....
Plaster	0 ....
Postoperative radiograph .	0 ....
Stay	1 day ....
Follow up	2 weeks ....

Operative requirements   Paediatric tourniquet.

Postoperative care
Babies do not need physiotherapy and they will start to
use the thumb after the discomfort from the operation
has settled.

Complications   Division of a digital nerve to the thumb.

Operation: release of trigger finger in an adult

The first annular (A1) pulley, which forms the entrance
to the flexor sheath, is divided through a 1 cm transverse
incision, just beyond the distal palmar crease. If performed under LA the patient should be able to flex and
extend the digit with the wound open and demonstrate
that it no longer triggers.

Codes

GA/LA	GA or LA ....
Blood	0 ....
Antibiotics	0 ....
Time	20 minutes ....
Drains	0 ....
Plaster	0 ....

Postoperative radiograph .. 0 ....

Stay .... Day case ....

Follow up .... 2 weeks ....

Off work .... Depends on occupation ..

**Operative
requirements**   Tourniquet.

Management   **Postoperative care**
Encourage the patient to use the finger immediately.

Complications   Division of a digital nerve.

33 De Quervain's stenosing tenovaginitis

The condition
De Quervain's is due to impingement of and synovitis around, the tendons of extensor pollicis brevis and abductor pollicis longus in their canal over the radial styloid.

Making the diagnosis

The patient   The patient is usually a middle-aged female.

The history   The patient complains of pain just proximal to the anatomical snuff box, which worsens on using the hand.

On examination   There may be a palpable swelling over the tendons.
On active flexion and extension of the thumb you may be able to feel crepitus in the first dorsal compartment.
Finkelstein's manoeuvre may be used to confirm the diagnosis. This is performed by holding the thumb adducted in the palm whilst flexing the hand in ulnar deviation. This will reproduce the pain.

Treatment
If the symptoms are only of a few weeks' duration, an injection of steroid into the canal, around the tendons, may be curative.

Indications for surgery   Persistent symptoms that have not responded to conservative therapy.

Operation: decompression of de Quervain's tenovaginitis
A longitudinal incision is made over the tendons. The roof of the canal is divided. Care must be taken to see and preserve the superficial branches of the radial nerve.

Codes

GA/LA	GA . . . .
Blood	0 . . . .
Antibiotics	0 . . . .
Time	½ hour . . . .
Drains	0 . . . .
Plaster	0 . . . .
Postoperative radiograph .	0 . . . .
Stay	Day case . . . .
Follow up	10 days . . . .
Off work	10 days . . . .

Postoperative care

Management

Elevate the hand for the first day postoperatively.
Encourage use of the thumb immediately.

Complications

Failure to completely divide the entire sheath may lead to persistent symptoms.

Division of the superficial radial nerve may leave an anaesthetic area on the dorsum of the thumb and also produce a painful neuroma.

The condition

This is a contracture of the palmar aponeurosis that leads to a gradually increasing flexion deformity of the affected finger.

Making the diagnosis

The patient   The typical patient is a middle-aged male. He may be of Celtic descent, with pale blue eyes and fair hair. There may be a family history of the disease. The commonly stated association between Dupuytren's and alcoholism is probably spurious. There is a high incidence in epileptics receiving phenytoin therapy and in diabetics.

The history   The patient will either complain of a painful nodule in the palm, or of a painless thickening in the palm and the inability to straighten his finger. The latter typically leads to the finger getting caught when putting his hand in his trouser pocker and to poking himself in the eye when washing his face!

On examination   Examine both hands.

Carefully document the location of the fascial bands. They are over the flexor tendons in the palm, but go to one or other side of the tendon as they enter the finger.

Make a note of the range of movement in the metacarpophalangeal, proximal interphalangeal and distal interphalangeal joints in each of the affected fingers.

If the patient has had previous surgery, note the position of the scars and examine the sensation in the finger to see if the digital nerves are still intact.

Ask the patient to put his hand flat on the table and see if the diseased finger prevents him laying the hand completely flat.

Treatment

Indications for surgery   Surgery is indicated if the contracture prevents the palm being laid flat on the table. In severe cases where the tip of the finger is embedded in the palm, amputation of the finger may be the best option.

The patient must be warned that contracture of the proximal interphalangeal joint is usually associated with a secondary flexion contracture of the joint itself. Thus the joint cannot usually be fully extended, even when the Dupuytren's bands are excised.

The patient must be warned of the risk of digital nerve injury.

Operation: partial (palmar) fasciectomy for Dupuytren's contracture

Zig-zag skin incisions are used with the apices at the skin creases of the joints. This is done to avoid the risk of a joint contracture that would occur if a straight incision was used that subsequently contracted.

The abnormal fascial bands are then carefully dissected free and removed. The digital nerve is especially at risk as it wraps around the band at the level of the metacarpophalangeal joint.

If there is a skin contracture, one can either perform Z-plasties to gain extra skin length, or the wound can be left open and allowed to close secondarily (McCash open palm technique).

Codes

GA/LA	GA
Blood	0
Antibiotics	0
Time	1–2 hours
Drains	Yes
Plaster	0
Postoperative radiograph	0
Stay	3 days
Follow up	2 weeks
Off work	4 weeks

Operative requirements   High arm tourniquet.

Management

Postoperative care

Elevate the hand whilst an in-patient.

Check the sensation in the distribution of the digital nerves at risk.

Beware haematoma. Hand operations are not generally painful postoperatively — if the patient complains of severe pain, remove all of the dressings and inspect the wound. If there is a haematoma, removal of one or two sutures may be enough to allow its evacuation. If this fails, the patient may have to return to theatre to have the haematoma drained.

If the wound has been drained, the drain can usually be removed after 24 hours.

The surgeon should take down the dressings and check that the skin flaps are viable after 48 hours postoperatively, prior to discharging the patient.

Complications

Division of a digital nerve.

Postoperative haematoma.

Death of a skin flap.

Residual contracture of the proximal interphalangeal joint.

Divided flexor tendons

The condition

This is a common injury. The injury to the tendons may be accompanied by division of the neurovascular bundles.

The zone of injury between the distal interphalangeal joint and the palm, where the tendons run in the flexor canal, is known as 'no-man's land'. Following surgery, adhesions can prevent smooth gliding of the tendon in the canal and this accounts for the difficulty in achieving good results from tendon repair in this zone.

Making the diagnosis

The history

The patient may have a laceration that is quite small. Establish the exact mechanism of injury. If the fingers were flexed whilst receiving the cut, as in someone who grasps a knife blade, the tendon ends will be some distance from the original wound when the fingers are in extension. This latter position is how the fingers will be on the operating table and may make retrieval of the tendon ends difficult.

On examination

Look at the hand at rest. The fingers normally lie slightly flexed, but if the flexor tendons are divided the finger will lie extended.

Examine the function of the superficial flexor and the deep flexor for each finger:

(a) hold the patient's fingers extended that are *not* being examined. Ask the patient to flex the finger that is free. The superficial flexor tendon is intact if he flexes the finger at the proximal interphalangeal joint;

(b) to examine the deep flexor tendon, hold the proximal interphalangeal joint in extension of the finger being examined. Then ask the patient to flex the tip of the finger. Deep flexor function is intact if the patient can flex the distal interphalangeal joint;

(c) a normal variation in the little finger is the inability to flex the proximal interphalangeal joint whilst the other fingers are held extended. If there is a possibility that a flexor tendon to the little finger has been cut, compare the injured with the uninjured side.

Examine sensation in the fingers and ensure that they have an intact vascularity with good capillary refill at the fingertips.

Radiographs Radiographs of the hand are essential to exclude a fracture or the presence of a foreign body.

Preoperative management

Common associated injuries Divided digital nerve or artery.

Preparation for surgery Clean and then dress the wound with a saline-soaked swab.

If the interval until operation is likely to be more than a few hours, immobilize the hand in a back-slab up to the fingertips, with the wrist and the metacarpophalangeal joints flexed. This may reduce the retraction of the cut tendons.

Give tetanus toxoid if the patient is not fully covered.

Treatment

Indications for surgery Laceration in the hand with a clinical suspicion of a flexor tendon injury.

Contra-indication to surgery Late presentation, i.e. after more than 48 hours, with a contaminated wound. In these patients, it is better to let the wound heal and perform the exploration as an elective, delayed procedure, 10 days or more after the injury.

Operation: repair of divided flexor tendons in the hand

The laceration is extended in a zig-zag fashion with the apices of the incision at the skin creases of the joints.

This avoids the risk of a joint contracture that would occur if a straight incision was used that subsequently contracted. Once retrieved, the tendons are repaired using a meticulous technique to diminish the risk of adhesions within the tendon sheath and a subsequently poor result.

Codes

GA/LA	GA ....
Blood	0 ....
Antibiotics	Yes ....
Time	1 hour ....
Drains	0 ....
Plaster	Below elbow ....
Postoperative radiograph .	0 ....
Stay	2 days ....
Follow up	1 week ....
Off work	6 weeks ....

Operative requirements

High arm tourniquet. The operating microscope should be available in theatre if there is a likelihood of a digital nerve or artery repair.

Postoperative care

Management

Mobilization instructions depend on whether dynamic traction with elastic bands, or passive mobilization is used. Some surgeons place an elastic band on the fingertip which goes to a pulley over the wrist. This allows the patient to extend the finger actively and then for the finger to be flexed passively by the elastic band and not the repaired tendons (Kleinert traction). Others instruct the patient on exercises where active extension is permitted, but the patient uses their other hand to flex the injured finger. These regimes of early movement prevent the development of adhesions when the tendon repair is within the tendon sheath.

If a digital nerve has also been repaired, the finger has to remain flexed for 3 weeks, but passive mobilization can be continued.

Complications   Injury to neuro-vascular bundle in the digit.
Infection.
Stiffness.
Rupture of repaired tendon.

36 Infection in the hand

The condition

Pus may be localized in the midpalmar and thenar spaces in the hand, or may track along the tendon sheaths from a finger into the palm and wrist.

Making the diagnosis

The history

The patient may have had a minor puncture wound that initially went unnoticed. They may be in an occupation that is at risk for infection.

The patient will complain of increasing pain in the hand that may become excruciating. The patient may be systemically unwell.

Ask about a family history of diabetes, as this infection may be the first presentation of the disease.

On examination

The patient's temperature must be measured.

If the infection is in a deep space in the hand, the hand will be swollen, red and exquisitely tender. Due to the unforgiving nature of the palmar fascia, the swelling may be maximal on the dorsum of the hand.

With a tendon sheath infection the affected finger will be red, swollen and held flexed. Any movement of the finger, either actively or passively, will be exceedingly painful. You must examine the palm and the wrist for tenderness. This is because the infection may track down the tendon sheath. In the thumb and the little finger, the sheath is continuous with the bursae in the wrist. The sheaths of the middle three fingers open into the palm.

Radiographs

Order radiographs of the hand and fingers to exclude a foreign body or underlying osteomyelitis.

Preoperative management

Investigations

These must include a full blood count and ESR. If the patient's pyrexia is greater than 38°C, take blood cultures.

If you are at all suspicious of the infection being the first presentation of diabetes, measure the blood glucose.

Preparation for surgery

Rest the hand in a back-slab and elevate.

Treatment

Indications for surgery

A localized collection of pus that is not draining spontaneously.

Tendon sheath infection.

Operation: incision and drainage of hand infection

For a palmar space infection, the incision is made directly over the abscess. For a tendon sheath infection, a lateral incision is made in the fingertip and a transverse one in the palm, so that the tendon sheath can be irrigated.

Codes

GA/LA	GA . . . .
Blood	0 . . . .
Antibiotics	Start after a specimen of pus has been obtained . . . .
Time	½ hour . . . .
Drains	0 . . . .
Plaster	Below-elbow volar-slab up to fingertips . . . .
Postoperative radiograph .	0 . . . .
Stay	3–4 days . . . .
Follow up	2 days . . . .
Off work	2 weeks . . . .

Operative requirements

Have a tourniquet on the upper arm, but try to avoid its use. If a tourniquet is used, exsanguinate the limb by elevation only. Send a specimen of pus for immediate Gram stain and culture. Once the specimen has been taken, start intravenous flucloxacillin+/– Fucidin until the sensitivities are available. If the entry wound was due to a punch injury from an opponent's teeth, add metronidazole.

Postoperative care

Management
    Immobilize the whole hand in a volar-slab with the metacarpophalangeal joints at 70 degrees, and the proximal interphalangeal and distal interphalangeal joints extended, until the infection has completely resolved.

    Elevate the upper limb.

    Obtain microbiology results as soon as possible and if necessary, change the antibiotic regime.

Complications
    Inadequate drainage and debridement resulting in re-accumulation of pus.

Fractured metacarpal

The condition
The metacarpal may fracture at the neck, through the shaft or at the base.

Making the diagnosis

The history   A punch, falling onto a clenched fist or a direct blow are the usual causes of a metacarpal fracture. The patient will complain of pain and swelling around the fracture.

It is important to know the dominant hand and the occupation of the patient. The age is also a consideration, as one may accept displacement in an 80 year old that you would not in a 20 year old.

On examination   It is vital that you look for a rotational deformity. This is best done by asking the patient to slowly flex the fingers. If pain inhibits active flexion by the patient, you should passively and gently flex the fingers. If there is no rotational deformity, all the fingers will point toward the scaphoid, without over- or underlapping. Always compare the injured hand with the normal hand.

Examine the distal circulation of the injured finger (capillary refill) and look for evidence of a nerve injury.

Radiographs   The whole hand.

Preoperative management

Preparation for   Immobilize the hand in a below-elbow volar-slab, with
surgery   the metacarpophalangeal joints at 70 degrees and the fingers straight.

Treatment
Undisplaced fractures and those with acceptable angulation on the lateral view do not require anything more than immobilization for 2–3 weeks. The amount of acceptable angulation increases from 15

degrees for the index metacarpal to 30 degrees for the fifth metacarpal.

Simple transverse or oblique fractures may need closed manipulation and the insertion of percutaneous K-wires.

More comminuted fractures may need open reduction and internal fixation.

Indications for surgery

A rotational deformity is an absolute indication for surgery. If there is considerable shortening of the metacarpal, especially of the index finger, surgery is often necessary.

Operation: metacarpal fracture — 1 closed reduction and K-wiring, 2 open reduction and internal fixation

1 Under image intensification, the fracture is reduced and then held with one or two K-wires passed percutaneously. It is often simplest to pass the wires transversely through into the adjacent metacarpal. The wires are left with their ends exposed to allow them to be removed on follow up in the clinic.

2 The fracture is reduced through an incision on the dorsum of the hand. It is then held with either screws alone, or with screws and a plate.

Codes

GA/LA	GA or regional block ....
Blood	0 ....
Antibiotics	Yes ....
Time	1 hour ....
Drains	0 ....
Plaster	Yes ....
Postoperative radiograph .	AP and lateral hand .....
Stay	2 days ....
Follow up	2 weeks ....
Off work	6 weeks ....

Operative requirements

Mini-fragment AO set or K-wire set.
Tourniquet.
Image intensifier and radiographer.

Management

Postoperative care

Elevate the hand until discharge the next day.

The duration of plaster immobilization depends on the rigidity of the fixation and must be specified by the surgeon. Ideally the fixation should be rigid enough to start immediate, gentle, active mobilization.

Complications

Infection.

Loss of position.

Reduced range of movement of the finger due to adhesion of the extensor tendons to the plate.

38 Ruptured ulnar collateral ligament of the thumb (gamekeeper's thumb)

The condition
Injury to the ulnar collateral ligament of the meta-carpophalangeal joint of the thumb may be a sprain or a complete rupture. Originally described as an overuse laxity in gamekeepers, the term 'gamekeeper's thumb' is nowadays used to describe an acute injury.

Making the diagnosis

The history
This injury results from sudden dorsiflexion and abduction of the thumb. It is common after a fall on a dry ski slope, where the thumb gets caught in a hole in the mat, or during a fall whilst snow skiing when the thumb is wrenched by the strap of the ski pole.

The patient will complain of pain around the meta-carpophalangeal joint at the base of the thumb. They may also have noticed a weakness in pinch grip. This is due to the lack of stability of the metacarpophalangeal joint of the thumb.

On examination
There is pain and tenderness around the ulnar side of the metacarpophalangeal joint. With the metacarpal fixed by the examiner, a complete rupture will be demonstrated by the fact that the joint opens on being stressed.

Make sure that you examine the other thumb to establish the normal laxity of the ligament and the normal range of flexion of the metacarpophalangeal joint for that patient.

Radiographs
Radiographs of the thumb may show a bone fragment avulsed from the ulnar corner of the proximal phalanx. If the diagnosis is in doubt, stress films can be taken comparing the two thumbs.

106

Treatment

If the ligament is sprained, or the fracture of the base of the proximal phalanx is undisplaced, the thumb is immobilized in a plaster cast for 4 weeks.

Indications for surgery

Complete rupture of the ulnar collateral ligament, or avulsion of its insertion with the bone fragment being displaced.

Operation: open repair of ulnar collateral ligament of the thumb

The joint is exposed through a dorso-medial incision over the joint.

If the bone fragment is big enough, it may be held with a mini-fragment screw. If it is too small, a suture is passed through the ligament into the proximal phalanx.

If the ligament is ruptured in its mid-substance, the two ends are sutured together. If the rupture is old, it may be necessary to use a tendon graft from palmaris longus to reconstruct the ligament.

Following repair, the joint may be immobilized by a K-wire.

Codes

GA/LA	GA . . . .
Blood	0 . . . .
Antibiotics	Optional . . . .
Time	¾ hour . . . .
Drains	0 . . . .
Plaster	Thumb spica . . . .
Postoperative radiograph . .	AP and lateral MCP joint only if bone fixed . . . .
Stay	2 days . . . .
Follow up	4 weeks . . . .
Off work	6 weeks . . . .

Operative requirements

Mini-fragment AO set or small K-wire set.
Tourniquet.

Management

Complications

Postoperative care
Elevate the hand whilst an in-patient.
The plaster is kept on for a minimun of 3 weeks.

Division of dorsal branch of the radial nerve.
Stiff metacarpophalangeal joint.

39   Bennett's fracture-dislocation of the thumb

The condition

This is a fracture of the base of the first metacarpal that is intra-articular.

Making the diagnosis

The history

The injury occurs following violent extension of the thumb. The injury may occur following a fall or during a contact sport such as rugby. The patient will complain of pain just distal to the anatomical snuff box.

On examination

There is usually pain and tenderness around the base of the metacarpal. You may feel instability and crepitus on extending the thumb.

Radiographs

Request AP and lateral radiographs of the metacarpophalangeal joint of the thumb. The palmar corner of the base of metacarpal remains in place on the trapezium. If the fracture is displaced, the rest of the metacarpal is dislocated dorsally from the trapezium.

Treatment

If the fracture of the base of the first metacarpal is truly undisplaced, it is not a Bennett's fracture-*dislocation* and the thumb can be immobilized in a scaphoid-type plaster cast. If there is a dislocation, it must be reduced and then held.

Indications for surgery

As this is an intra-articular fracture, accurate reduction is required. This may be possible by closed manipulation, with the fracture being held with a K-wire passed percutaneously. If this is unsuccessful, an open reduction is performed and the position held with K-wires.

Operation: Bennett's fracture-dislocation of the thumb — 1 manipulation under anaesthesia +/− K-wiring, 2 open reduction and K-wiring

1 Under screening with the image intensifier, it may be

possible to reduce the fracture closed and hold the position with a padded cast. If not, the position can be held with K-wires passed percutaneously.

2 If closed reduction is not successful, a dorsal incision is made over the base of the metacarpal. The fracture is reduced and held with K-wires.

Codes

GA/LA...............	GA or regional block ....
Blood	0.....................
Antibiotics	Yes, if open reduction ...
Time.................	1 hour ....
Drains...............	0.....................
Plaster...............	Scaphiod cast ....
Postoperative radiograph .	AP and lateral thumb ....
Stay.................	48 hours ....
Follow up	1 week, X-ray on arrival ..
Off work	6 weeks ....

Operative requirements
Image intensifier and radiographer.
K-wire set and powered driver.

Postoperative care

Management
The arm should be elevated for the first 24 hours.
K-wires are removed after 5 weeks, in the clinic.

Complications
Failure to achieve anatomical reduction.

Spinal Column

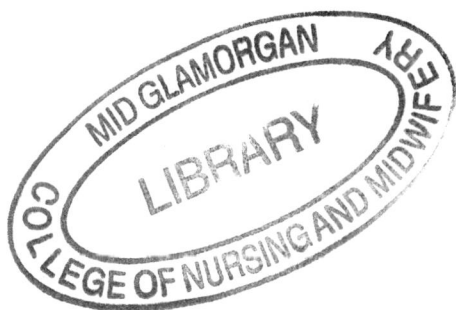

40

Fracture of a cervical vertebra

The condition
Fractures of the cervical vertebrae include:
1 Flexion or extension injuries where the only bony abnormality is a small piece of bone avulsed from the upper or lower anterior borders of the vertebral body.
2 A major fracture that includes the posterior elements and is unstable.
3 A fracture with retropulsion of fragments into the bony canal resulting in injury to the spinal cord.
4 A fracture of the odontoid peg that is unstable.
One or both facet joints at a single level may dislocate without a fracture.

Making the diagnosis

The patient
A patient who is conscious with a significant neck injury, will have severe pain in the neck and spasm of the paracervical muscles. Such a patient is relatively safe from suffering further injury, due to this protective spasm.

Any unconscious patient who has had significant trauma of any type, especially a blow to the head, must be presumed to have an unstable cervical spine injury until proved otherwise. If there is such an injury, the unconscious patient lacks protective spasm and further damage to the spinal cord can occur if the neck is not kept immobilized.

The history
Cervical fractures are common after direct trauma, such as diving into a shallow pool. They can also occur with indirect trauma such as the rapid flexion and extension that occurs in a head-on collision with another car.

On examination
On a conscious co-operative patient, gently examine the *active* range of the movements of the neck — flexion/ extension, lateral flexion and rotation — and express them as a percentage of those of a normal person. Perform a complete neurological examination of the

upper and lower limbs, i.e. sensation, motor power, reflexes, and plantar responses. Check the patient's rectal tone and perianal sensation.

Radiographs

The minimum view that is acceptable is a lateral of the whole cervical spine. The C7/T1 junction *must* be seen. This may require someone to pull down on the patient's arms to draw down the shoulders whilst the radiograph is taken, or a swimmer's view (with the arm nearest the X-ray tube extended above the head) or even lateral tomograms.

If flexion and extension views are required to exclude instability, they should only be performed on an awake co-operative patient. A doctor should supervise the examination, which must be discontinued if the patient has any abnormal symptoms, such as tingling in the upper or lower limbs.

If a facet dislocation or unstable fracture is suspected, oblique views are required followed by either lateral tomograms or a CT scan or both.

Preoperative management

Prior to definitive management, the neck must be immobilized with a well-fitting stiff collar.

Treatment

If the fracture is stable, immobilization in a well-fitting stiff collar is often adequate.

If there is a fracture that is unstable but is in an acceptable position, the spine must be immobilized. This can be achieved by either skull traction, a halo-vest or a Minerva jacket.

If there is significant displacement of a fracture or an unstable injury, this must be reduced either by traction, by manipulation under anaesthesia or by open operation. Once reduced, the position must be maintained until healing has occurred.

Indications for skeletal traction

An unstable neck fracture or a facet dislocation in an adult.

**Contra-
indications to
skeletal traction**

Children and the very elderly, whose skulls are too soft.

Operation: application of skeletal skull traction

A simple and safe means of applying traction is with
'cone callipers'. The pins are inserted 2.5 cm (1 in.) above
the top of the ear. Alternatively, a halo can be used as a
means of traction allowing the addition of the vest later
on. The sites for the pins are infiltrated with local
anaesthetic down to and including the periosteum,
and shaving of the hair is not necessary. The pins are
designed so as to prevent penetration of the inner table
of the skull.

Codes

GA/LA	LA ....
Blood	0 ....
Antibiotics	0 ....
Time	½ hour..............
Drains	0 ....
Plaster	0 ....
Postoperative radiograph .	See below ....

**Operative
requirements**

Skull traction can be applied in the casualty department.
Local anaesthetic (lignocaine and adrenaline).
Two doctors.
Complete set of traction equipment.
Traction bed.

Postoperative care

Management

For fractures — 2.25 kg (5 lb) traction.
For a facet dislocation, start with 2.25 kg (5 lb) traction
and obtain a radiograph as soon as the patient is in
traction. If still dislocated, increase the weight immediately by 0.5–1 kg (1–2 lb) and obtain a repeat radiograph within the hour. Repeat this increase in weight,
followed by a repeat radiograph, until the dislocation

is reduced. Once reduced, decrease the traction to 2.25 kg (5 lb).

Complications   The inner table of the skull may be perforated with excessive torque, a pathologically porotic skull or misplaced pins and a subsequent pin tract infection can lead to meningitis.

41

Acute low back pain

The condition

The cause of acute low back pain is often obscure. However, the majority are due either to a muscle sprain, or local facet joint disease, or to a prolapsed intervertebral disc.

A prolapse of an intervertebral disc usually occurs as an acute event accompanied by the onset of severe sciatica (pain down the back of the leg in the distribution of the sciatic nerve). The disc prolapse is usually lateral but may be central. This rare central disc protrusion does not necessarily produce sciatica but may press on the nerves supplying the sacral plexus and cause irreversible damage to bowel and bladder function.

The investigation of a patient with severe back pain without sciatica must exclude inflammatory causes such as ankylosing spondylitis, external pressure on the vertebrae such as an aortic aneurysm, and bony disease that may be benign or malignant, primary or secondary.

Making the diagnosis

The patient   Acute low back pain and disc prolapse typically occurs in adults between 20 and 40 years. Elderly patients do not usually suffer disc prolapse as discs become desiccated with ageing.

The history   Find out if there have been preceeding episodes of pure back pain prior to the disc prolapse. These may represent weakening of the annular ligament which then ruptures, giving rise to the disc prolapse.

Ask what percentage of the pain is from the back and what percentage is from the leg.

Establish whether the sciatica radiates down to, or below, the knee.

What makes the leg pain worse? Of note is laughing, coughing, sneezing, or straining at stool. All of these are associated with an increase in intradural pressure.

Is there any bladder or bowel dysfunction?

What pain killers does the patient take and how often?
Does the pain wake the patient or prevent him from sleeping?

On examination   The examination must include a general examination to exclude a primary malignant disease.

Perform a complete neurological examination of the lower limbs.

Look for signs of nerve root irritation, i.e. a limited straight-leg raise that produces sciatica which increases with dorsiflexion of the ankle, or internal rotation of the hip or pressure on the popliteal nerve. A crossed-leg sign (sciatica when the contralateral straight-leg raise is performed) is also a reliable indicator of a disc protrusion.

Do not omit a rectal examination. Lack of perianal sensation and poor rectal tone may indicate a central disc protrusion. This is rare, but is a surgical emergency and must be decompressed as soon as possible to preserve bladder and bowel function.

Radiographs   AP and lateral views of the lumbo-sacral spine (these are invariably normal in a patient with a disc protrusion).

Preoperative management

Investigations   If the cause of the back pain is not clinically obvious, then a screen for possible causes should be performed. This should include the following:

Chest radiograph.

Full blood count.

ESR.

Urea and electrolytes.

Blood glucose.

Liver function tests.

Calcium and alkaline phosphatase.

Serum immunoelectrophoresis.

Radioisotope bone scan.

If there are signs of a nerve root compression this can be confirmed on a radiculogram and/or a CT scan, or an MRI scan.

Treatment

Conservative treatment

For an acute, severe episode of back pain, including patients who clinically have a prolapsed disc, the initial treatment is always *strict* bed rest. The decision to admit the patient depends on the home circumstances of the patient and the severity of their pain.

Prescribe a strong analgesic, such as aspirin and papaveretum, to be taken regularly rather than p.r.n. Ensure that the patient does not become constipated — back pain and constipation are an unpleasant combination. Also prescribe a non-steroidal anti-inflammatory.

As an adjunct to instructions for bed rest, the patient can be placed on either pelvic traction via a harness with 7.2 kg (16 lb) weight, or skin traction with 2.25 kg (5 lb) on each leg. When symptoms diminish after about 1 week, the patient should be mobilized with the help of the physiotherapist.

Remember that 90% of patients with back pain will improve without any major intervention.

Indications for surgery

The patient may be helped by a caudal epidural injection of steroid if they have either:

Back pain and sciatica, but a myelogram that does not correlate with the clinical findings.

Persistent leg pain following disc surgery.

Disc excision and nerve root decompression is indicated for the patient with *all* of the following:

Severe leg pain that has not improved after several weeks of conservative treatment.

A disc prolapse that is proven on a myelogram or CT scan.

Clinical features which are consistent with the abnormal level of the radiological investigations.

Contraindications to surgery

Back pain with minimal leg pain.
Improving symptoms.

Procedure: radiculogram (lumbar myelogram)

A water-soluble radio-opaque 'dye' is injected into the

cerebro-spinal fluid via a spinal needle. The nerve roots are outlined and compression of the nerves shows up as a filling defect in the column of contrast. A specimen of cerebro-spinal fluid is sent to microbiology for microscopy, culture and sensitivity, and to chemical pathology for estimation of the protein content. After the plain films have been taken, a CT scan of the abnormal levels, with the contrast still in place, may reveal additional information.

Indications

Sciatica and the clinical features suggestive of a prolapsed intervertebral disc.
Symptoms of spinal stenosis (see Chapter 42).
Possible spinal tumour.

Contra-indications

Back pain without leg pain.
A patient who will not consider surgery even if the radiculogram shows nerve root compression.

Codes

GA/LA	LA . . . .
Blood	0 . . . .
Antibiotics	0 . . . .
Time	1 hour . . . .
Stay	Day case or overnight . . . .
Follow up	10 days . . . .
Off work	3 days . . . .

Requirements

Since a radiculogram is an invasive procedure with some risks, the patient has to give signed consent. In many hospitals it is the house officer rather than the radiologist who has to obtain it.

Management

Postoperative care

The postradiculogram instructions are usually provided by the radiologist. The patient is encouraged to drink fluids, is kept on bed rest for 12 hours but allowed to sit up at 30 degrees.

Complications   Postmyelogram headache. If this occurs, rest the patient in bed and prescribe a mild analgesic. The patient should remain in hospital until comfortable enough to go home. Although the headache usually occurs within 24 hours, it can start after the patient has left the hospital and the patient should be warned of this.

Operation: caudal epidural injection

A caudal injection of a cocktail of local anaesthetic, steroid and saline is introduced into the epidural space via the sacral hiatus. The success rate is only 70% and it may take some weeks before there is any improvement.

Codes

GA/LA	GA
Blood	0
Antibiotics	0
Time	¼ hour
Drains	0
Plaster	0
Postoperative radiograph	0
Stay	Day case
Follow up	12 weeks
Off work	2 days

Operative requirements   The injection can be performed in the anaesthetic room.

Postoperative care

Management   The patient may become hypotensive in the first few hours after the epidural injection. This should be treated with elevation of the foot of the bed and the administration of intravenous fluid.

The patient should commence back exercises immediately.

Complications   Hypotension.
Acute retention of urine.
No improvement in symptoms.

Operation: excision of prolapsed intervertebral disc (discectomy/fenestration/laminectomy)

The extradural space is entered through a midline posterior incision. Generally only the ligamentum flavum needs to be removed, but if this gives an insufficient view, part of the lamina is removed — a fenestration. In the past, the whole lamina was removed, hence it was known as a laminectomy. If the operating microscope is used, the incision is considerably smaller and the operation is known as a micro-discectomy.

If the disc is actually prolapsed, the pieces that lie outside the annulus but under the posterior longitudinal ligament are removed. If the disc is bulging without having prolapsed completely, the posterior ligament and the annular ligament are incised and the disc material removed from the disc space. This can be hazardous, as the anterior relation to the anterior longitudinal ligament is the aorta. There have been cases where a hole has been made in the aorta, with fatal consequences!

The patient must be aware that the aim of the operation is to remove leg pain and prevent permanent neurological deficit in the leg. Its purpose is *not* to cure back pain, which may remain postoperatively.

Codes

GA/LA	GA
Blood	Group and save
Antibiotics	Yes
Time	1½ hours
Drains	0
Plaster	0
Postoperative radiograph	0
Stay	10 days
Follow up	6 weeks
Off work	2–3 months

Operative requirements

The patient is generally operated upon in the prone position. However, some surgeons prefer the patient to be in the lateral position with the side to be explored uppermost. This does have the advantage that blood runs out of the wound, rather than pooling at the bottom.

For a micro-discectomy, the image intensifier is used to ascertain the correct level prior to making the skin incision. For a non micro-discectomy, a plain radiograph is occasionally required to check the level. Ask the surgeon if this is his practice, so that you can arrange for the radiographer to be in theatre.

Postoperative care

Management
The house officer must check that the patient is neurologically intact immediately postoperatively.

Mobilization regimes vary from surgeon to surgeon. In general, when the patient can arch their back and perform a straight-leg raise, they can get out of bed and be mobilized by the physiotherapist.

No heavy lifting for at least 6 months.

Complications
Temporary or permanent damage of the nerve root. This would give an isolated muscle group and dermatome deficit — *not* paraplegia as many patients imagine.

Dural tear — if this is not sealed at operation, a persistent leak can lead to the formation of a CSF fistula.

Extradural haematoma — this gives a cauda equina syndrome and requires urgent decompression.

Wound infection.

Persisting leg pain.

Discitis — infection in the disc space.

Operating on the wrong level, leading to persistent symptoms and further surgery at the correct level.

Spinal instability.

The condition

In spinal stenosis there is narrowing of the bony spinal canal that may be due to hypertrophy of the posterior disc margin, osteophytes on the facet joints and infolding of the ligamentum flavum. The stenosis may also be due to a degenerative spondylolisthesis. This is a slippage forward of one vertebra on the one below, with resultant narrowing of the bony canal. Spinal stenosis can be congenital as in achondroplastic dwarfs.

Making the diagnosis

The patient   The patient is usually elderly.

The history   The patient complains of pain and/or heaviness, that comes on with exercise, in both legs or occasionally only one leg. The pain diminishes when the patient rests with the spine flexed, e.g. leaning forwards. This story is often confused with vascular claudication.

On examination   A full general examination should be performed.

A complete neurological examination of the lower limbs must be performed. Look for signs of nerve root irritation. You may be able to reproduce the symptoms by exercising the patient. In addition, an ankle jerk that was present prior to the exercise, may be absent after exercise.

Check that the lower limb pulses are present to exclude a true vascular cause for the symptoms.

Radiographs   The lateral view of the lumbosacral spine will show a spondylolisthesis if present.

A CT scan is the best method of demonstrating the cross-sectional area of the bony spinal canal. However, a narrowing in the column of contrast in a radiculogram can also be diagnostic.

Treatment

Indications for surgery
Severe symptoms and radiological confirmation of spinal stenosis.

Operation: decompression of spinal stenosis

The bone and ligament which are compressing the dura are excised through a midline posterior incision. The number of levels that are decompressed depends on the findings on the CT scan and the radiculogram. If, after an extensive decompression, the surgeon feels that the spine may have been made unstable, an intertransverse fusion is performed at the same time.

Codes

GA/LA	GA . . . .
Blood	Group and save . . . .
Antibiotics	Optional . . . .
Time	1½ hours . . . .
Drains	0 . . . .
Plaster	0 . . . .
Postoperative radiograph .	0 . . . .
Stay	10 days . . . .
Follow up	6 weeks . . . .
Off work	3 months . . . .

Operative requirements
The patient is operated upon in the prone position. If an intertransverse fusion is planned at the same operation as the decompression, you must include on the consent and the theatre list that a posterior iliac crest bone graft is to be taken.

Postoperative care

Management
The patient is mobilized as comfort allows.

Elderly patients often go into urinary retention and if a urethral catheter is necessary, it should be left in until the patient is mobile.

A reflex ileus is not uncommon, so ensure that bowel sounds are present before allowing the patient to eat and drink.

If there has been a dural tear, the patient should be kept on bed rest for 2–3 weeks to try and prevent fistula formation.

Complications   Temporary or permanent damage of the nerve root. This would give an isolated muscle group and dermatome deficit — *not* paraplegia as many patients imagine.

Dural tear — if this is not sealed at operation, a persistent leak can lead to the formation of a CSF fistula.

Extradural haematoma — this gives a cauda equina syndrome and requires urgent decompression.

Urinary retention.

Paralytic ileus.

Wound infection.

Discitis — infection in the disc space.

Persistent leg pain.

43   Back pain associated with spinal instability

The condition

There is abnormal movement between one or more vertebral bodies. A spondylolisthesis is a forward slip of the vertebra above on the one below. This may be due to:

1 Spondylolysis — a defect in the pars interarticularis that may be familiar or the result of a stress fracture.

2 Spondylosis — degenerative changes in the facet joints.

3 Postoperative instability following an extensive laminectomy.

Making the diagnosis

The history

The patient complains of back pain that is well localized. The pain is usually intermittent, coming on after exercise. Take a full history that includes the duration, nature, site, radiation and exacerbating factors of the pain. Ask about bowel and bladder function.

On examination

Perform a complete neurological examination of the lower limbs which should include the following tests:

(a) ask the patient to heel walk and toe walk, this demonstrates muscle weakness (or lack of it) around the ankle;

(b) compare the straight-leg raise with the patient sitting on the edge of the bed and lifting each leg in turn, with the straight-leg raise with the patient lying flat.

Inconsistency between the two examinations of the straight-leg raise may be an indicator of psychological overlay.

Do not omit a rectal examination.

Radiographs

The minimum required are recent AP and lateral views of the lumbo-sacral spine. It may be necessary to have lateral views in flexion and extension to see abnormal

127

movement between the adjacent segments. If nerve root involvement has to be excluded, a radiculogram and/or a CT scan may be required. If the spondylolisthesis is due to a spondylolysis, oblique views of the lumbar spine may be needed to show the bony defect of the pars interarticularis.

Preoperative management

Operative requirements

In general an iliac crest bone graft is taken and consent for this is vital.

The patient will be operated upon in the prone position, and the anaesthetist should be informed of this so that a guarded endotracheal tube is inserted.

Treatment

Indications for surgery

Persistent back pain with a demonstrated, progressive slip.

Operation: intertransverse fusion/alar-transverse fusion

The incision may be a midline posterior incision, two separate parallel paravertebral vertical incisions, or a single horizontal incision. The spinal canal is not exposed unless the fusion accompanies a spinal decompression. Cancellous bone for grafting is taken from the posterior iliac crest. The transverse processes are exposed and decorticated. Bone graft is laid upon the transverse processes and the gap in between. The facet joints have their articular cartilage removed and then bone graft is inserted into the joints to fuse them.

If the fusion is between adjacent lumbar vertebrae it is termed 'intertransverse'. If the fusion is between the transverse processes of L5 and the ala of the sacrum, it is called an alar-transverse fusion.

Codes ·

GA/LA...............	GA ....
Blood	2 units ....
Antibiotics	0 ....
Time.................	1½ hours ....

Drains	Yes . . . .
Plaster	(Rarely) hip spica . . . .
Postoperative radiograph .	0 . . . .
Stay	10 days . . . .
Follow up	6 weeks . . . .
Off work	2–3 months, depending on occupation . . . .

Postoperative care

Management

The patient stays on bed rest until he is able to bridge (i.e. arch the back).

Urinary retention is common postoperatively and if a catheter is inserted, it should be left in for a few days, until the patient is able to get out of bed. However, you must ensure that the retention is not neurologically based, by checking that the patient has the feeling of a full bladder and has normal perianal sensation and rectal tone.

A reflex ileus is not uncommon, so ensure that bowel sounds are present before allowing the patient to eat and drink.

The patient may be immobilized in a plaster hip spica but this is not common. If used, the plaster is applied after 5 days postoperatively and is kept on for 5 weeks.

Complications

Urinary retention.

Deep vein thrombosis.

Failure of fusion.

Persistence of back pain, even if the fusion is solid.

Persistent pain from the iliac crest bone graft donor site.

The condition
Vertical force through the spine leads to loss of height of a vertebra, typically at the L1 level. In the young this requires considerable force. In the elderly osteoporotic female, it may be the result of a trivial fall.

In the young, the bone is more resistant to compression, so the vertebra tends to spread and fragments of bone may be pushed into the spinal canal. These may press on the spinal cord and give neurological problems. However, surprisingly large fragments of bone may lie in the canal without any clinical neurological deficit.

In the elderly it is almost always a stable injury.

Making the diagnosis

The history
In the young, there will be a history of a fall from a height with the patient landing either on their feet or their backside. The patient will have severe pain at the level of the crushed vertebra. He may have other fractures and you should ask about heel pain in particular.

The elderly patient will have a history of a stumble or gentle fall. However the pain may be quite severe and may be enough to incapacitate the patient so that admission becomes necessary.

On examination
Log roll the patient (with help from the nurses) and examine the back for the site of tenderness and for any gibbus (a prominence due to a forward angulation in the spinal column.)

Check bowel and bladder function, including a rectal examination.

Perform a full neurological examination of lower limbs.

Radiographs
Obtain good quality AP and lateral views of the lumbar spine. If there are doubts about the stability of the spine, a CT scan may be required.

Initial management

Treat the patient as having an unstable fracture until definitely disproved. This means log rolling the patient in order to turn them, and avoiding flexion and extension.

Preoperative management

Common associated injuries

Calcaneal fractures.

Treatment

For the elderly, all that is required is for the patient to be on bed rest for a few days whilst the pain settles. They are then gently mobilized in a corset with the help of the physiotherapists.

In the younger patient who has no abnormal neurological findings and an anterior compression which is less than 50% of the height of the vertebral body, treatment is bed rest for 6 weeks, followed by mobilization in a plaster or plastic jacket.

Indications for surgery

An unstable fracture.

A fracture with fragments of bone in the spinal canal (seen on the CT scan) and a deteriorating neurological deficit.

Young patients with greater than 50% loss of vertebral height.

Operation: decompression of the spinal canal and Harrington rod stabilization

The spine is approached posteriorly. If indicated, the bony canal is opened and the bone fragments removed.

Harrington rods with sublaminal hooks are used to distract and thus reduce the fracture. One rod is placed on each side of the spinous processes and they are attached to broad hooks that are slipped under the edges of the laminae. The instrumentation is fixed to the two vertebra above and the two below the vertebra that is fractured.

Codes

GA/LA................	GA ....
Blood	4 units ....
Antibiotics	Yes ....
Time..................	2 hours ....
Drains.................	Yes ....
Plaster.................	0 ....
Postoperative radiograph..	AP and lateral lumbar spine ....
Stay...................	2 weeks ....
Follow up	6 weeks ....
Off work	3 months ....

Postoperative care

Management Once the spine has been stabilized, the patient is safe to be mobilized as the pain allows. Urinary catheterization is often required postoperatively.

Complications Neural damage that may include making an incomplete neurological lesion complete.
Infection.
Late pull out of a sublaminal hook.

45   Pelvic fracture (excluding pubic rami fracture of the elderly)

The condition

A fracture of the pelvis is the result of considerable energy and is often found in a patient with multiple injuries.

Rupture of the venous plexus in the pelvis can lead to massive internal haemorrhage. A patient with a displaced pelvic fracture can exsanguinate without a drop of blood being lost onto the bed!

Making the diagnosis

The history

One needs to know the exact mechanism of injury. If the patient was in a road traffic accident, was he/she the driver of the vehicle? Was he/she wearing a seat belt? At what speed did the impact occur?

Take a history that does not concentrate on the obvious injury. You need to know about the patient's general health, etc. You also need to know where else he hurts.

Ask whether or not the patient has passed urine spontaneously since the injury.

On examination

Examine the whole patient, as the force required to fracture a pelvis can damage other bones or viscera.

Examine the perineum for bruising.

Look for blood at the urethral meatus which may signify a urethral injury.

If one leg is shortened, this is likely to be due to a hip dislocation.

Examine the neuro-vascular status of the lower limbs. Loss of an ankle jerk may be due to sciatic nerve damage.

Radiographs

An AP view of the pelvis is the only view that should be obtained in the resuscitation room.

If the fracture involves the acetabulum, ask for Judet views (iliac and obturator obliques) which show up the anterior and posterior columns of the acetabulum.

133

These are not required urgently and can be obtained when the patient is stable.

The pelvis is a ring. If there is a fracture that is displaced, there must be another discontinuity in the ring. Always remember to look at the sacro-iliac joints to see if they are intact.

A CT scan of the pelvis is often required to determine the exact configuration of the fracture. If a hip dislocation has been reduced, a CT scan will show whether or not fragments of bone remain in the joint or if there is a femoral head fracture.

Preoperative management

Investigations

Full blood count.

Urinalysis for haematuria.

Common associated injuries

Cervical spine injury, long bone fracture, ruptured urethra, torn bladder and abdominal injury.

Treatment

Emergency treatment

Pelvic fractures bleed internally, so make sure that there is adequate venous access (two 14 gauge cannulae) and adequate fluid and blood replacement (6 units minimum).

If the patient has not passed urine, consider the possibility of a urethral injury. Gently try passing a urethral catheter. Do not use force, as there is the risk of making an incomplete urethral tear complete. If there is any difficulty, insert a suprapubic catheter.

If the hip is dislocated, it must be reduced under a general anaesthetic and a femoral traction pin inserted. If the fracture involves the acetabulum or there is gross displacement of one side of the pelvis, a femoral traction pin should be inserted in the casualty department, using local anaesthetic.

If the pelvic fracture is of the open-book type, the application of an external fixator and closure of the 'book' may help reduce the blood loss.

Definitive treatment

A patient with an undisplaced extra-articular fracture is treated with bed rest for 6 weeks.

An extra-articular pelvic fracture which is unstable needs to be stabilized, either with an external fixator or by open reduction and internal fixation.

Undisplaced and minimally displaced acetabular fractures are usually treated with skeletal traction.

Displaced acetabular fractures need accurate reduction, stable internal fixation and early motion.

Operation: acetabular fracture; insertion of a femoral Denham or Steinmann pin for skeletal traction +/− manipulation under anaesthesia of dislocated hip

If the hip is dislocated posteriorly, as is common, it is reduced by one person pressing down on both anterior superior iliac spines, whilst a second person flexes the hip to 90 degrees and then pulls up.

A Denham pin (which is threaded in its mid part) or a Steinmann pin (which is smooth) is inserted across the distal femur and 6.75 kg (15 lb) of traction is added.

Codes

GA/LA	GA or LA if pin insertion alone . . . .
Blood	6 units . . . .
Antibiotics	0 . . . .
Time	½ hour . . . .
Drains	0 . . . .
Plaster	0 . . . .
Postoperative radiograph . .	AP pelvis and Judet views
Stay	6 weeks . . . .
Follow up	6 weeks . . . .
Off work	3 months minimum . . . . .

Operative requirements
Steinmann/Denham pin insertion pack. If the hip needs to be reduced, one or two strong assistants are of great help.

Postoperative care

Management
Apply 6.75 kg (15 lb) of skeletal traction.

Monitor the pulse, blood pressure and urine output at least hourly for the first 24 hours.

Complications   Exsanguination!
Hip dislocation.
Urethral injury.
Associated intra-abdominal injury, e.g. splenic rupture.

The condition

A fractured pubic ramus is a common minor injury in the elderly.

In a younger patient, a pubic ramus fracture is a serious injury and must be treated as a major pelvic fracture (see Chapter 45).

Making the diagnosis

The history

An elderly woman will have had a minor fall and present with pain in the hip and the inability to weight bear. The history often leads one to initially suspect a fracture of the femoral neck.

On examination

The leg will *not* be short or externally rotated. Examination of the range of movements of the hip may cause some discomfort.

Radiographs

An AP of the pelvis will show the fracture of one or both pubic rami. If a patient has a lot of hip pain with a radiograph that looks normal, it may be worth obtaining a bone scan. This may highlight a pubic ramus fracture that has not been appreciated previously.

Preoperative management

Common associated injuries

In the elderly, any fracture associated with osteoporosis.

Treatment

The patient is admitted for bed rest and should be prescribed oral analgesia. When the pain settles the patient should be mobilized.

Codes

Blood	0 . . . .
Plaster	0 . . . .
Stay	10–14 days . . . .
Follow up	6 weeks . . . .

Complications   Those of an elderly patient confined to bed, i.e. deep vein thrombosis, urinary tract infection, pressure sores, respiratory tract infection.

Lower Limb

The condition

The incidence of congenital dislocation of the hip is 2.5 per 1000 live births. Dislocation is more common in girls and the left hip is more often affected than the right.

The risk factors are:

A family history of congenital dislocation of the hip.

Breech delivery.

The presence of a foot deformity.

Any other congenital abnormality.

Making the diagnosis

The patient

A dislocatable or dislocated hip may be diagnosed when the newborn baby is examined for this and other disorders.

Alternatively, the diagnosis may not be made until the child begins to walk and a limp is noticed.

On examination

With a hip which is dislocated (as opposed to dislocatable) the buttock skin creases are asymmetrical and the leg is slightly shortened.

Abduction is limited compared to a normal newborn baby whose flexed hips should abduct so that the legs end up flat on the couch.

Ortolani's sign is positive if there is a palpable clunk when the hip is abducted, reducing the dislocated hip.

Barlow's test is positive if downward pressure along the femur, with some lateral force, makes a reduced hip dislocate.

In the older child with a dislocated hip, Trendelenburg's sign is positive and there is a Trendelenburg gait.

Radiographs

Radiographs before the child is 6 weeks old are of little value as the head of the femur has not ossified. After the head begins to ossify, but before it has done so completely, dislocation is inferred by abnormalities in lines drawn onto the AP view of the pelvis.

Preoperative management

Investigations
Ultrasound of the hip is becoming increasingly popular to identify abnormal hips in the newborn. The advantage is that structures that are not visible on a plain radiograph can be identified by non-invasive means.

An arthrogram of the hip gives information about the congruence of the hip which can be easily interpreted. Radio-opaque contrast is injected into the hip joint and is seen with the image intensifier. Unlike an ultrasound, an arthrogram has to be performed under a general anaesthetic.

Treatment

A newborn with a dislocatable hip, or a hip that is dislocated but can be reduced, is nursed in double nappies or an abduction harness for 6 weeks. The majority of these are normal at their 6-week review.

A child with a dislocated hip that cannot be reduced by Ortolani's test, is placed in gallows traction (legs suspended vertically in skin traction) and the legs are gradually abducted to full abduction over 2 weeks. If, with the hips fully abducted, the hip is fully located, the child is placed in a plaster cast that includes both hips, for 6 weeks. The child is then kept in a splint that prevents adduction but allows some movement, for a further 10 months.

If, after gradual abduction in gallows traction, the hip remains dislocated, an open reduction is performed.

At open reduction the hip may only be stable with the femur in internal rotation and abduction. If so, the child is placed in a plaster with the leg in the appropriate position for 6 weeks. Then an upper femoral osteotomy is performed to maintain the reduction.

Indications for surgery
A child who is less than 6 years old with a dislocated hip that cannot be reduced by conservative mehods.

Operation: open reduction of congenital dislocation of the hip

The hip is approached via an anterior incision. The

structures preventing reduction of the hip are removed from the joint and the hip is reduced.

Codes

GA/LA	GA . . . .
Blood	Group and save . . . .
Antibiotics	0 . . . .
Time	1½ hours . . . .
Drains	0 . . . .
Plaster	Hip spica . . . .
Postoperative radiograph .	AP pelvis . . . .
Stay	5 days . . . .
Follow up	6 weeks . . . .

Operative requirements

An on-table arthrogram is usually performed prior to open reduction. Theatres and the radiographer need to the informed beforehand.

Postoperative care

Management

The hip spica cast is kept on for 6 weeks. If necessary, an upper femoral osteotomy is then performed.

Complications

Avascular necrosis of the femoral head.

Operation: upper femoral osteotomy in a child

The child is operated upon on an ordinary operating table with a sand-bag under the hip. A lateral incision is made. The upper femur and anterior femoral neck are exposed and the osteotomy performed. The osteotomy is held with a nail plate.

Indications for surgery

This operation is performed on children and has several indications:

Following open reduction of a congenitally dislocated hip.

Acetabular dysplasia, with 'uncovering' of the femoral head.

Excessive femoral neck anteversion resulting in intoeing.

Codes

GA/LA	GA . . . .
Blood	Group and save . . . .
Antibiotics	Yes . . . .
Time	1½ hours . . . .
Drains	0 . . . .
Plaster	0 . . . .
Postoperative radiograph .	AP pelvis and lateral hip . .
Stay	7 days . . . .
Follow up	6 weeks . . . .
Off work	3 weeks . . . .

Operative requirements

Check with the surgeon and specify on the operating list, what type of nail plate is to be used.

A radiolucent operating table should be used, in case an intraoperative check radiograph is necessary.

Postoperative care

Management

The child is allowed up with the help of crutches when the immediate postoperative pain has settled. It is impossible to restrict a child's weight bearing and they should be allowed to do whatever is comfortable.

The plate and screws are removed after 1 year.

Complications

Wound infection.

Incorrect orientation of osteotomy.

The condition

This is a non-specific condition that affects young children. Its significance is that serious causes of hip pain have to be excluded before making the diagnosis of an irritable hip. One must exclude septic arthritis, Perthes' disease, slipped upper femoral epiphysis and tuberculosis.

Making the diagnosis

The patient   The child is usually aged between 4 and 9 years old and will have had no previous hip complaints.

The history   The child complains of an increasing pain in the hip and is unwilling to walk. There may be a history of the child having recently had a cold or 'flu.

On examination   The child is generally well, without a fever. The child will either have a limp or simply refuse to walk. On examination of the hip, all movements will be painful, but the discomfort is worst at the extremes of movement. Extension of the hip is normally the movement which is most severely restricted (and the last to be regained).

Radiographs   One must obtain a radiograph of the hip to exclude infection, Perthes' disease and slipped upper femoral epiphysis. By definition, the radiograph is normal in the irritable hip.

Management

Investigations   Blood must be taken for a full blood count and erythrocyte sedimentation rate. If the child is very young and you are not practised at drawing blood from children, ask the paediatricians for their help.

Consider obtaining a Heaf test and a chest radiograph if the child is from a community where tuberculosis is not uncommon.

Treatment

A child who is unable or unwilling to weight bear must
be admitted, placed on bed rest, with 2.25 kg (5 lb) of
skin traction on the affected leg. After 4 or 5 days,
the hip should be more comfortable and the child can
be allowed up. Keep the child in hospital until they
are completely recovered with a full, pain-free, range
of movement.

The child must be followed up for a minimum of
3 months. This is in case the irritable hip was a
preliminary to the development of Perthes' disease.

The condition

The epiphysis of the femoral head can 'slip' off the neck. This may be a gradual or a sudden process. It is not common.

Making the diagnosis

The patient

The patient is usually between 10 and 15 years old. It is more common in boys. The patient is typically fat with poor secondary sexual development. There may be a demonstrable hormone imbalance or deficiency, e.g. hypothyroidism, but this is rare.

The history

A history of specific trauma is rare. The child may complain of increasing hip pain but often the pain may be referred to the knee. (Beware the 10-year-old boy with knee pain — examine the hip!) If the slip is acute-on-chronic, there will a history of mild hip pain which suddenly worsens.

On examination

The patient will often have a limp. When the slip has occurred, the leg will be short and externally rotated. All movements of the hip may be uncomfortable, but the most significant signs are limited internal rotation and limited abduction.

Radiographs

Most slips are visible on an AP view of the pelvis. A line drawn up the superior edge of the neck of the femur should pass into the head of the femur. If the line passes outside the head, the head has slipped. The posterior edge of the acetabulum should cut across the medial corner of the upper femoral metaphysis. It does not do so when the epiphysis has slipped. If there is any doubt about whether or not the epiphysis has slipped on the AP view, ask for frog lateral views of both hips.

Preoperative management

Investigations

Consider hypothyroidism.

Preparation for surgery

Whilst waiting for surgery, the child may be more comfortable with 2.25 kg (5 lb) of skin traction on the affected leg.

Treatment

Indications for surgery

All slipped epiphyses require fixation *in situ*.

Even a severe slip should not be manipulated into a better position prior to fixation. This is because the manipulation may further damage the already injured blood supply to the femoral head, resulting in avascular necrosis.

There is debate whether or not to prophylactically pin the contralateral hip, as bilateral slippage is common (25%).

Operation: internal fixation of slipped upper femoral epiphysis

With the child on the orthopaedic table, a small lateral incision is made down to the greater trochanter. The pins are inserted up the femoral neck into the femoral head. The position of the pins is checked with the image intensifier. With a severe slip, the head may be so far backwards that the entry point for the pins may be quite anterior on the neck.

Codes

GA/LA	GA
Blood	2 units
Antibiotics	Yes
Time	1 hour
Drains	0
Plaster	0
Postoperative radiograph	AP pelvis and lateral hip
Stay	1 week
Follow up	6 weeks
Off school	4 weeks

Operative requirements

The requirements are the same as when inserting a dynamic hip screw, i.e. image intensifier and radiographer.

The surgeon should specify the type of implant to be used.

Management

Postoperative care

Full blood count at 48 hours.

Encourage the child to mobilize the hip and knee whilst in bed.

When the pain subsides the child is allowed up, non-weight bearing with crutches.

Complications

Poor fixation leading to further slippage.

Attempted reduction can lead to avascular necrosis of the femoral head.

Penetration of the pin through the articular cartilage of the femoral head may cause pain on movement of the hip and damage to the articular cartilage.

The condition

Osteoarthritis of the hip may be primary, or secondary to trauma or to previous joint disease.

Rheumatoid arthritis frequently results in the destruction of the hip joints.

Making the diagnosis

The patient

Patients who present for a joint replacement are usually over 60 years, but not always. Patients with rheumatoid arthritis may be much younger.

The history

Ask about predisposing factors including family history, hip problems as a child (sepsis, congenital dislocation of the hip, Perthes' disease and slipped upper femoral capital epiphysis) and trauma. Inquire as to the state of the other major joints, especially if the patient is known to suffer from rheumatoid arthritis. It is important to know which joint is causing the patient most distress.

When taking the specific history of the hip pain, you should establish:

The severity and any radiation of the pain.

Whether or not the pain wakes the patient at night.

What analgesics the patient takes and how often.

Whether or not the patient is able to put their shoes and socks on normally.

Whether or not the patient is able to cut their own toe nails.

How the patient goes up stairs? Normally, or by placing both feet on each step, holding onto the bannister?

If the patient uses a stick indoors or just outdoors.

Whether or not the patient has a limp.

Take a social history that includes the patient's occupation, hobbies, home circumstances, e.g. stairs, and whether or not the patient lives alone.

On examination

Watch the patient walk. Note any limp and whether they use a stick.

Look for scars from previous operations around the hip.

Perform Trendelenburg's test to test for weak abduction.

Note any fixed flexion deformity with Thomas's test.

Examine the range of flexion, abduction and adduction of both hips. Examine external and internal rotation with the hips extended.

Look for apparent shortening and measure true shortening.

Check that the foot pulses are present.

Check that there are no abnormal neurological findings in the lower limb.

Do not omit a rectal examination of the prostate from the examination of a male patient.

Radiographs   Ensure that there is a recent AP view of the whole pelvis and a lateral view of the diseased hip.

If the patient has rheumatoid arthritis (with neck symptoms), obtain AP and lateral views of the cervical spine to exclude instability.

Preoperative management

Investigations   Midstream urine.

Preparation for surgery   Most surgeons like their patients to have a shower or bath, washing with an antiseptic soap, the night before and on the day of surgery.

Treatment

The initial treatment for all arthritic joints is medical. This includes analgesics and anti-inflammatory drugs, as well as physiotherapy. The use of a walking stick and a non-steroidal anti-inflammatory drug may be enough to relieve the pain of many patients.

Indications for surgery   A total hip replacement is indicated for either osteo-arthritis or rheumatoid arthritis of the hip if it is accompanied by severe pain. It is also indicated for failed fixation of a subcapital hip fracture.

A total hip replacement may fail because of either deep infection or loosening. If at all possible, the hip replacement is renewed. However, this may not be possible and the patient may be left with a Girdlestone's excision arthroplasty.

Contra-indications to total hip replacement

Minimal symptoms, however bad the radiographic changes.

Ischaemic heart disease or peripheral vascular disease that would obscure the benefits of hip replacement; i.e. if the angina or claudication is so severe that the patient would still not be able to walk very far following surgery, the risks may outweigh the benefits.

Urinary tract infection.

Prostatism that may result in postoperative urinary retention and the need for a prostatectomy. It is better to have the urological investigations and surgery *before* a total hip replacement.

Operation: total hip replacement

The hip can be approached through a variety of routes. The postero-lateral, the lateral and the antero-lateral are the three common approaches.

Once exposed, the hip is dislocated. The acetabulum is prepared by removing the remaining articular cartilage and some of the cortical bone. The femoral head and part of the neck are removed and the femoral canal is prepared so as to take the stem of the component.

Hip replacements generally have a metal femoral stem with a metal head, that articulates with a high density polyethylene acetabular cup. The acetabular component may be totally plastic or may be metal backed.

The components may be held with bone cement that contains barium so that it is visible on the radiographs. The cement may also contain an antibiotic. Remember that cement is not a glue and works by its interdigitation rather than adhesion.

Alternatively, one or both components may be inserted 'uncemented', with the femoral stem being a press fit, and the acetabulum being either a press fit or held by screws or pegs. The lack of cement has the advantage of making subsequent revision surgery easier, but the disadvantage of having an initially poorer fixation. Uncemented components are often used for younger patients (under 60 years), since the likelihood of needing a revision is high. At best, a hip replacement may last 15–20 years, but sometimes it may last less than 5 years.

Codes

GA/LA...............	GA or spinal ....
Blood	4 units ....
Antibiotics	Yes ....
Time.................	2 hours ....
Drains...............	Yes ....
Plaster...............	0 ....
Postoperative radiograph ..	AP whole pelvis and lateral hip ....
Deep vein thrombosis prophylaxis	Yes ....
Stay.................	10–14 days...........
Follow up	6 weeks ....
Off work	3 months.............

Operative requirements

State on the operating list exactly what prosthesis is to be used and whether or not it is cemented.

Postoperative care

Management

Check that the femoral nerve and the sciatic nerve are intact. Ask the patient to press their knee into the bed. If the quadriceps tighten, the femoral nerve is intact. If the patient can wiggle their toes and has sensation in the foot, the sciatic nerve is undamaged.

Remove the drains by the second postoperative day.

Check haemoglobin on postoperative day 2.

If the patient does not pass urine and has to be catheterized, you must give him/her an appropriate antibiotic whilst the catheter is in place.

The regime for mobilization depends upon the surgical approach and whether the components are cemented or uncemented:

(a) If uncemented components have been implanted, the patient is usually kept partial weight bearing with crutches for 2–3 months.

(b) In general, the posterior approach to the hip requires that the patient should avoid sitting up for 3–5 days. During this time the patient should go straight from bed to standing. Anterior and lateral approaches to the hip are more stable with the hip flexed than the posterior approach and so the patient can sit in a chair immediately.

(c) Since the posterior approach is potentially unstable in adduction and internal rotation, the patient's locker is kept on the same side of the bed as the operated leg and the patient is advised to sleep on their back for 3 months following surgery. This is because, as the patient rolls onto their side, the upper leg falls into adduction and internal rotation, whereas the lower leg stays in neutral. If the patient cannot tolerate sleeping on their back, then they may sleep on the operated side with a pillow between the legs.

Many patients ask about when they can be allowed to drive:

(a) In general a patient will usually regain their preoperative reaction time by 2 months postoperatively and is then safe to drive.

(b) If they drive an automatic car and the left leg has been operated upon, they can drive sooner than if it was the right leg.

(c) It is the patient's ultimate decision whether or not they feel safe to drive.

Complications

Injury to nerves and vessels.
Intraoperative femur fracture.
Wound infection.
Deep vein thrombosis and pulmonary embolism.
Loosening of one or both components.
Infection of the prosthesis.

Operation: revision of total hip replacement

This is a considerably more difficult operation than a primary hip replacement. The exposure has to be more extensive and the soft tissue dissection greater.

If loose, removal of the components themselves is easy. However, removal of the bone cement from the femoral shaft can be a painstaking and laborious task. As the cortex is often thinner than normal, there is the dual risk of either perforating the shaft and/or breaking it. Special cement-removing instruments are needed and a special revision prosthesis may be required. Autogenous or banked bone may be needed to fill defects.

If the original prosthesis is being removed for infection, the revision is usually performed in two stages. At the first operation, the infected components are removed, samples of tissue and fluid are sent for microbiological examination and beads containing an antibiotic are left in the wound. The second operation is after 6 weeks treatment with the appropriate antibiotics, when the new prosthesis is inserted.

Codes

GA/LA...............	GA ....
Blood	6 units ....
Antibiotics	Yes ....
Time..................	2–4 hours............
Drains................	Yes ....
Plaster................	0 ....
Postoperative radiograph ..	AP pelvis and lateral hip .
Deep vein thrombosis prophylaxis	Yes ....
Stay..................	2 weeks ....
Follow up	6 weeks ....
Off work..............	3 months.............

Operative requirements   Cement-removing instruments.
The theatre list should state if one or both components

are to be revised, what design/make is being removed and what type is going to be inserted.

If only one component is to be removed, the femoral head must be of the same circumference as the inner diameter of the acetabular cup, so look in the notes to see what size was originally used. Common head sizes are 22 mm, 28 mm and 32 mm.

If a long-stemmed femoral component is anticipated as being necessary, ensure that it is available.

Postoperative care

Management

The intraoperative and postoperative blood loss can be considerable. You must check on the amount of drainage in recovery, on the evening of the first day postoperation, and the next morning. The amount of blood replaced should nearly equal the amount of total blood lost.

Check that the femoral nerve and the sciatic nerve are intact. Ask the patient to press their knee into the bed. If the quadriceps tighten, the femoral nerve is intact. If the patient can wiggle their toes and has sensation in the foot, the sciatic nerve is undamaged.

If the arthroplasty seemed a little unstable on the operating table, the patient may need to remain on bed rest for longer than usual or may even require skeletal traction.

Due to the greater tissue dissection, patients who have had a revision hip take longer to mobilize than after a primary total hip replacement. Otherwise the mobilization instructions are similar to those given for a primary hip replacement.

Complications

The complications associated with primary hip surgery are all more common after revision surgery:
Injury to nerves and vessels.
Intraoperative femoral fracture.
Dislocation.
Deep vein thrombosis and pulmonary embolism.
Infection of the prosthesis.
Loosening of one or other components.

The condition

A total hip replacement is most at risk of dislocating in the immediate postoperative period that commences with the patient being moved off the operating table onto their bed. In the first days and weeks, the muscles are weak and there is no scar tissue around the new joint. It is during this time that most care must be taken.

The position in which a total hip replacement is most unstable partly depends on the surgical approach that was used when the prosthesis was inserted. Following the posterior approach, the hip is most at risk when flexed, adducted and internally rotated. Following the antero-lateral and the lateral approaches, the hip is most unstable in extension with external rotation.

More than one dislocation may indicate malposition of one or both components and the prosthesis may need to be revised.

Making the diagnosis

The history

When taking the history, you must find out exactly what the patient was doing and what position the leg was in when the hip dislocated, especially if it has occurred more than once.

On examination

If the hip has dislocated posteriorly, the leg lies shortened, flexed and internally rotated. If the dislocation is anterior, the leg lies extended and externally rotated.

Radiographs

Ask for an AP and a lateral view of the hip.

Treatment

If the hip is very unstable, it may be possible to relocate the joint under intravenous sedation. However, it is usually safer to give the patient a general anaesthetic.

Operation: reduction of dislocated total hip replacement

The hip is usually easily reduced by a combination of gentle traction and internal or external rotation. If the manipulation is performed in theatre, one should screen the hip under the image intensifier to establish the position of instability.

Codes

GA/LA...............	GA ....
Blood	0 ....
Antibiotics	0 ....
Time..................	10 minutes ....
Drains.................	0 ....
Plaster.................	Occasionally ....
Postoperative radiograph ..	AP and lateral hip ......
Stay..................	Depends on time since original operation .....
Follow up	6 weeks ....
Off work	6 weeks ....

Operative requirements   Image intensifier and radiographer.

Postoperative care

Management   If the patient is in the immediate postoperative period, the surgeon may decide to keep the patient on bed rest on traction for 6 weeks to allow the false capsule to form.

If the hip is unstable in flexion, the patient can have a plaster cylinder applied to keep the knee extended.

Complications   Recurrent dislocation.

Inability to reduce the hip closed, necessitating an open reduction.

52

Fractured neck of femur

The condition
This is commonly a fracture of the elderly and is due to osteoporosis. The proportion of elderly in the population is increasing, as is the age-specific incidence of the fracture. This will result in an exponential rise in the overall incidence of this fracture in the next 10–20 years.

Although these fractures are of the neck of the femur, they are commonly referred to as hip fractures.

The anatomical location of the fracture determines the treatment. The main differentiation depends on whether the fracture is intracapsular or extracapsular.

Intracapsular fractures result in the blood supply to the femoral head being put at risk. This is because the vessels which enter the bone at the base of the neck, at the site of attachment of the capsule, are the main source of blood supply to the femoral head. If an intracapsular fracture is reduced and internally fixed, the greater the original displacement, the greater the likelihood of either non-union of the fracture or of avascular necrosis of the femoral head. Although intracapsular fractures can be divided into subcapital, transcervical and basicervical, they are all referred to as subcapital fractures in general parlance.

Extracapsular fractures do not damage the blood supply to the femoral head, so they are all reduced and internally fixed.

Patients with a fractured neck of femur are associated with at least 30% mortality in the 6 months following surgery.

Making the diagnosis
The patient These elderly patients are often infirm and have multiple medical and social problems. It is these problems which usually prevent the patient's speedy return to their pre-injury abode.

The history

There will be a history of either a stumble or of the leg giving way.

The patient will have pain in the hip that prevents weight bearing.

A full history must be taken from either the patient or the care giver who may accompany the patient into hospital. If there is any doubt about past history or present medications, telephone the patient's general practitioner.

Establish the walking ability of the patient prior to the fall.

Ask about home circumstances. Does the patient live alone? If not, how fit is the spouse? Are there stairs up to the front door and/or inside? Does the patient have relatives or friends nearby?

If the patient lives in a nursing home, find out what level of activity is required before they can return to the home.

On examination

The injured leg is typically shortened, externally rotated and painful. Check the neurovascular integrity of the limb, especially the foot pulses.

Radiographs

Request an AP of the pelvis and a lateral view of the painful hip.

Intracapsular fractures are graded radiologically according to the Garden classification:

Garden I   Incomplete fracture through one cortex only

Garden II   Complete fracture running across the neck but without displacement

Garden III Complete fracture with partial displacement, with the femoral head adducted relative to the neck

Garden IV   Complete fracture with full displacement, so that the femoral head is translocated relative to the neck

Preoperative management

Preparation for surgery

Place 2.25 kg (5 lb) of skin traction on the injured leg.
If there is likely to be a delay in the patient being

operated upon, start an intravenous infusion. Many of the patients spend the night on the floor before being found and they may already be quite dehydrated prior to being kept nil by mouth whilst waiting for surgery.

Treatment

These fractures are operated upon to allow the patient to mobilize as quickly as possible and to try to avoid the complications of prolonged bed rest in the elderly.

Indications for surgery

Undisplaced or minimally displaced intracapsular (Garden grade I or II) hip fractures are fixed *in situ* using pins or screws.

In general, displaced intracapsular fractures are reduced and fixed in patients less than 70 years old. Reduction and internal fixation is contraindicated in patients who:

Are on steroid therapy.

Have poor mental health.

Have an interval between fracture and surgery greater than 48 hours.

The benefits of 'saving' the femoral head are in avoiding the complications of a hemiarthroplasty:

Pain in the hip, due to articulation of metal on cartilage.

Dislocation.

Infection.

Femoral fracture around the stem.

Acetabular erosion.

On the other hand, if the fracture unites, there is a 20–30% risk of avascular necrosis of the femoral head, which would then necessitate performing a total hip replacement.

In the older patient with an intracapsular fracture, the head of the femur is replaced by a hemiarthroplasty. The commonest prostheses used are the Austin–Moore, which is inserted without cement, and the Thompson's which is inserted with cement. Some surgeons use a 'bipolar' prosthesis.

Intertrochanteric hip fractures are reduced and then held with a dynamic hip screw, also known as a pin and plate.

Operation: dynamic hip screw for intertrochanteric fracture of the neck of femur

The patient is placed supine on the orthopaedic traction table with the feet in the traction boots. Ensure that the feet are well padded and secure. If they are not secure, they will pull out of the boots when traction is applied. The fracture is screened using the image intensifier and is reduced prior to any incision being made. A lateral incision is made down to the upper femur. A guide wire is passed up the neck of the femur under image intensifier control and the reamer for the screw passed over the guide wire. The lag screw is inserted up the neck and then the plate and barrel are applied to the femur and held with screws. As the fracture heals, it collapses and the sliding design of the screw within a barrel allows this to happen without the screw cutting out of the head. This is the 'dynamic' concept.

Codes

GA/LA	GA . . . .
Blood	2 units . . . .
Antibiotics	Yes . . . .
Time	1–1½ hours . . . .
Drains	Yes . . . .
Plaster	0 . . . .
Postoperative radiograph . .	AP pelvis and lateral hip .
Deep vein thrombosis prophylaxis	Optional . . . .
Stay	2 weeks minimum . . . . . .
Follow up	6 weeks . . . .

Operative requirements

Image intensifier and radiographer.
Orthopaedic traction table.

Management

Postoperative care
The patient is mobilized, fully weight bearing, as soon as the drain has been removed.

Check the haemoglobin on the second postoperative day.

Consider the social circumstances of the patient early and refer to social workers or geriatrician if necessary.

Complications
Wound infection.
Failure of fixation.
Chest infection.
Deep vein thrombosis.
Urinary tract infection.
Pressure sores.

Operation: internal fixation of subcapital fracture of the neck of femur

The patient is placed supine on the orthopaedic traction table with the feet held in the traction boots. Ensure that the feet are well padded and secure. The fracture is reduced under image intensifier control, prior to any incision being made.

A lateral incision is made down to the upper femur. Guide wires are passed up the neck of the femur under image intensifier control and the drill for the screws passed over the guide wires. Two or three screws are inserted up the neck and into the femoral head.

Codes

GA/LA	GA
Blood	2 units
Antibiotics	Yes
Time	1 hour
Drains	Yes
Plaster	0
Postoperative radiograph	AP pelvis and lateral hip .
Deep vein thrombosis prophylaxis	Optional
Stay	10–14 days
Follow up	6 weeks, X-ray on arrival

| Operative requirements | Orthopaedic table. Image intensifier and radiographer. |

Postoperative care

Management

Remove the drain after 24 hours.

The patient is mobilized out of bed after the drain has been removed.

Consider the social circumstances of the patient early and refer to the social workers or geriatricians if appropriate.

Complications

Deep vein thrombosis.

Pneumonia.

Urinary tract infection.

Congestive cardiac failure.

Failure of fixation.

Non-union.

Avascular necrosis of femoral head in 25%.

Operation: hemiarthroplasty for subcapital fracture of the neck of femur

The hip is approached through an antero-lateral or modified lateral approach. The fractured head is removed and replaced with a prosthesis. The most common types of prostheses used are the Austin–Moore hemiarthroplasty, which is used without cement, and the Thompson's hemiarthroplasty, which is used with cement. Some designs are known as bipolar. These have a small head articulating within a large shell. The aim of these designs is to reduce articulation at the true acetabulum and therefore reduce acetabular wear.

Codes

GA/LA .... GA ....

Blood .... 2 units ....

Antibiotics .... Yes ....

Time .... 1 hour ....

Drains .... Yes ....

Plaster .... 0 ....

Postoperative radiograph . AP pelvis and lateral hip . .

Deep vein thrombosis
prophylaxis. . . . .   Optional. . . . .
Stay . . . .   10–14 days . . . .
Follow up. . . . .   Optional. . . . .

Postoperative care

Management   Check haemoglobin on postoperative day 2.

Remove the drain after 24–36 hours.

Mobilize the patient after the drain has been removed, according to the surgical approach. The antero-lateral or lateral approaches allow the patient to sit up immediately, as they are stable with the hip flexed.

Cover urinary catheterization with an appropriate antibiotic.

Consider the patient's social circumstances early and if a problem is anticipated, refer to the social workers or geriatrician.

Complications   Deep vein thrombosis, pneumonia, urinary tract infection, congestive cardiac failure, etc.

Acetabular wear requiring later revision to a total hip replacement.

Dislocation.

Fracture of the femur at or below the tip of the prosthesis.

Pain on walking.

Fracture of the femoral shaft in a child

The history

Making the diagnosis

The diagnosis is usually obvious. It is important to know the mechanism of injury. If the child has been involved in a road traffic accident there may well be other significant trauma which must be looked for. It is all too easy to concentrate on the obvious injury. If the child has suffered a direct blow to the leg, then other trauma is unlikely.

In the toddler, always consider the possibility of the fracture being a non-accidental injury, but do not belabour the point.

On examination

Try and establish the diagnosis as quickly and painlessly as possible. Do not try and elicit crepitus at the fracture!

Check that the neurovascular status is intact distal to the fracture. This is vital so as to exclude a sciatic nerve injury.

Radiographs

Ensure that you have views of both the hip above and the knee below the fracture. Look to see if there is a concomitant hip dislocation or traumatic slippage of the capital epiphysis.

Common associated injuries

Preoperative management

Multiple injuries.
Hip dislocation.
Knee ligament injury.
Visceral injury.

Preparation for surgery

Make the child comfortable as soon as possible. As long as there is no significant head injury, give a single dose of intravenous morphine (0.125 mg/kg estimated body weight). Then insert a femoral nerve block using 0.5% bupivacaine hydrochloride (Marcain) in a dose 1.5 mg/kg estimated body weight. This will allow you to apply skin traction relatively painlessly.

Treatment

For a child who weighs less than 14 kg (30 lb), the definitive management is in gallows traction. This set-up has the child on his back, with both legs held vertically in skin traction. Enough weight is used to just lift the child's buttocks off the bed. The bandages must be removed daily to check on the condition of the skin, but the adhesive tape of the skin traction should not be disturbed. Once the fracture is 'sticky' and non-tender, a hip spica can be applied.

In a child who weighs more than 14 kg (30 lb), either longitudinal skin traction is used or 90/90 traction via a femoral traction pin.

When skin traction is to be used in conjunction with a Thomas' splint, determine the correct splint size by measuring the circumference of the thigh and the leg length of the uninjured side. Then fix on a Pearson knee flexion piece. The splint has to be set up for the appropriate side and it is usually up to the house officer to get the necessary bits and pieces. Use of the Thomas' splint also requires the house officer to check the splint daily and ensure that any pressure pads are correct in their pressure and location.

An alternative is Hamilton Russell traction, which combines below-knee skin traction with a sling placed under the knee. Due to the mechanics of the pulleys, 3 kg (7 lb) weight exerts 6 kg (12 lb) of traction on the leg.

Older children that are near to closure of their epiphyses, may need skeletal traction via a tibial traction pin and a Thomas' splint. The traction pin is placed lower than in an adult to avoid damaging the tibial apophysis. If necessary the insertion site can be checked with the image intensifier.

The position of the fracture must be checked with weekly radiographs for the first month and then monthly until the fracture is united.

Operation: insertion of tibial traction pin in a child

A Denham pin is inserted through the tibia below the level of the tibial apophysis under a general anaesthetic.

Codes

GA/LA	GA ....
Blood	Group and save ....
Antibiotics	Only if compound ....
Time	½ hour ....
Drains	0 ....
Plaster	0 ....
Postoperative radiograph .	AP and lateral femur in traction ....
Stay	1 week per year of age, max 12 weeks ....
Follow up.............	1 month, X-ray on arrival.

Operative requirements

The bed should be ready in theatre with all the traction set-up before the child is anaesthetized. This will enable the child to be placed in traction whilst still anaesthetized. It is up to the doctor to check that *everything* is correct. Never rely on anyone else.

Postoperative care

Management

Four and a half kilograms (10 lb) of traction should be applied initially. Take a check radiograph and adjust the traction accordingly. An overlap of 1.25 mm (0.5 in.) at the fracture is ideal, as the rate of growth of the femur increases following a fracture. If the fracture is brought out to length, this may result in the femur being too long after union of the fracture.

The pin sites should be wrapped and left undisturbed so long as they are not uncomfortable. Each ward sister, however, will have her own regimen for pin care.

Complications

Pin track infection.
Angular or rotational malunion.
Leg-length discrepancy.

54   Fracture of the femoral shaft in an adult

The condition

This common fracture is usually the result of a high energy injury. Therefore it may be found in a patient with multiple injuries.

Making the diagnosis

On examination

Try and establish the diagnosis as quickly and painlessly as possible. Do not try and elicit crepitus at the fracture!

Check that the neurovascular status is intact distal to the fracture by feeling the pedal pulses, checking sensation and asking the patient to move their toes. This is vital so as to exclude a sciatic nerve or femoral artery injury.

Examine the knee, as far as is possible, for bony or ligament injury. The force that fractured the femur may have passed via the knee and injured the latter in the process. A posterior cruciate rupture or a posterior hip dislocation is common after an injury where the knee has hit the dashboard with enough force to fracture the femur.

Radiographs

Ensure that the radiographs include views of both the hip above and the knee below the fracture. Look to see if there is a concomitant hip dislocation or fracture of the femoral neck. Look at the lateral view of the knee. Has the tibia fallen back, suggesting a posterior cruciate injury?

Preoperative management

Common associated injuries

Subcapital femoral neck fracture, hip dislocation or knee ligament injury.

Sciatic nerve injury.

Visceral injury.

Cervical spine injury.

Preparation for surgery

Make sure that there is good venous access — two size 14 cannulae — since closed femoral fractures can lose 4 units of blood into the thigh. In addition there may be an unrecognized injury that is associated with further blood loss.

Treatment

The initial management of a closed femoral fracture in an adult is skeletal traction via a tibial traction pin.

A femoral fracture may be treated conservatively with skeletal traction (for 3 months). Definitive management, however, is usually internal fixation with an intramedullary nail. If the fracture is open, an external fixator is commonly used.

In young adults, intramedullary nails are removed 18 months following their insertion. This is in case the patient injures the femur again and bends the nail, making it difficult or impossible to remove!

Operation: insertion of tibial traction pin in an adult

The pin is passed through the tibia 2.5 cm (1 in.) inferior and 2.5 cm (1 in.) posterior to the tibial tuberosity, entering on the lateral side. Anaesthetize the entry and exit sites with lignocaine. Use a hand drill to make the track through the tibia with a drill bit which is a little smaller than the Steinmann/Denham pin to be inserted. This will save on your sweat and the patient's pain.

Codes

GA/LA	LA
Blood	4 units
Antibiotics	Only if compound
Time	½ hour
Drains	0
Plaster	0
Postoperative radiograph	AP and lateral femur only if traction is definitive management

Operative requirements

A femoral nerve block can be used to reduce the pain from the fracture. Much of the discomfort associated with the pin's insertion is due to movement at the fracture site as the pin is pushed through the tibia.

If the pin is to be inserted in casualty, you need to borrow the Steinmann/Denham pin set, a hand drill and some drill bits from theatres. In addition, you need a suture pack, sterile drapes, local anaesthetic, skin prep. and sterile gloves.

Two people are required, one to actually insert the pin, and the other to hold the leg firmly and give counter pressure.

Management

Postoperative care

Skeletal traction is used to keep the patient comfortable until definitive surgery is performed. The traction is set up as the surgeon chooses. Four and a half to seven kilograms (10–15/lb) of traction is usually adequate. Traction can be simply straight to a pulley at the end of the bed or the leg may be elevated on a Thomas' splint.

Complications

Pin tract infection.

Operation: intramedullary nail for fractured shaft of femur

In the past a K (Küntscher) nail was used. Nowadays, an intramedullary nail is used that can be 'locked' with cross screws (AO nail, G–K or Grosse–Kempf nail, Russell Taylor nail). The nail can be locked proximally, or distally, or both.

The use of these locking screws depends on the level of the fracture in relation to the isthmus. The isthmus is the narrow midportion of the femoral shaft.

A fracture proximal to the isthmus needs to be locked proximally, as the nail will only have a good grip in the distal fragment.

A fracture distal to the isthmus needs to be locked distally, as the nail will only have a good grip in the proximal fragment.

If the fracture is at the isthmus or is comminuted, the

nail can be locked at both ends to prevent shortening or rotation.

The nail is usually inserted 'closed'. That is to say that the fracture itself is not opened and the procedure is monitored with image intensifier. With the patient on a traction table, traction is applied to a femoral traction pin and the fracture reduced. An incision is made in the buttock down to the tip of the greater trochanter. A guide wire is passed down the medullary cavity and across the fracture. Reamers are passed over the guide wire to enlarge the medullary cavity. The nail is then passed over the guide wire. If the nail is to be locked, screws are inserted across the nail, one proximally and/or two distally.

Codes

GA/LA	GA
Blood	3 units
Antibiotics	Yes
Time	1½ hours
Drains	Yes
Plaster	0
Postoperative radiograph	AP and lateral (whole) femur
Stay	10 days
Follow up	6 weeks
Off work	6 weeks

Operative requirements
Fracture table.
Image intensifier and radiographer.
A femoral traction pin, if not already in skeletal traction.

Postoperative care

Management
Check the haemoglobin on the second postoperative day.
Encourage hip, knee and ankle movement immediately.
If the fracture fixation is stable, the patient is allowed to mobilize fully weight bearing. If unstable, the patient can be mobilized non-weight bearing between crutches.

If the nail is locked at both ends, the patient may need readmission after 6 weeks, for removal of the screws from one end or the other (often referred to as dynamization).

Complications

Making a simple fracture complex!
Rotational malalignment.
Fat embolism.
Infection.
Compartment syndrome of the thigh (rare).
Deep vein thrombosis.
Loss of position; either shortening or rotational.
Non-union.

Operation: removal of intramedullary femoral nail

The original incision in the buttock is reopened. The first manoeuvre is to find the end of the nail. This may be difficult if it was hammered well down and bone has grown over the entry site. Secondly, the extraction device has to be engaged in the nail and, lastly, the nail must be hammered out. A nail may be so well embedded as to make removal impossible. Removal of a nail can often take longer than its insertion.

Investigations

Make sure that there are recent radiographs of the femur which show union of the fracture and include the upper end of the intramedullary nail.

Codes

GA/LA	GA ....
Blood	Group and save ....
Antibiotics	Optional ....
Time	1 hour ....
Drains	Yes ....
Plaster	0 ....
Postoperative radiograph .	AP and lateral femur.....
Stay	2 days................
Follow up............	6 weeks ....
Off work	2 weeks ....

Operative requirements

The surgeon must have the correct instruments for extraction of the nail. Therefore the theatre staff must know *exactly* what kind of nail is to be removed — Küntscher, Grosse – Kempf, AO, Russell–Taylor, etc. — and if there are locking screws. If you are in doubt as to the type of nail, look at the old operation note.

Management

Postoperative care
The patient can be mobilized immediately, fully weight bearing.

Complications

Fracture not truly united.
Refracture during nail removal.
Refracture postoperatively.
Inability to remove the nail.

55   Pathological fracture of the femur

The condition

Metastases in the bone are common and are often found in the femur. They typically occur in the subtrochanteric region. The patient may present with pain alone or with a fracture.

Tumours that commonly metastasize to bone are bronchus, breast, prostate, thyroid, kidney and myeloma. Primary bone tumours are much less common.

Making the diagnosis

The history

The patient may have had slight pain in the hip or thigh for some time prior to the fracture. The pathological fracture is often the first presentation of the malignancy. If this is the case, a thorough history must be taken to try and establish the site of the primary. Also ask the patient if they have any other pains, as these may be due to further bony secondaries.

On examination

Perform a complete and thorough examination to see if there is an obvious primary tumour.

Radiographs

Obtain radiographs of the *whole* femur to ensure that there is not another lesion in the femur. An internal fixation device inserted with its tip at the level of an unrecognized lesion, may precipitate a subsequent fracture.

Investigations

The best screening investigations after the history and examination are:
Full blood count.
Erythrocyte sedimentation rate.
Urea and electrolytes.
Liver function tests.
Acid phosphatase.
Calcium and alkaline phosphatase.
Thyroid function tests.
Serum immunoelectrophoresis.

175

Chest radiograph.
Bone scan.

Preparation for surgery

Preoperative management
In the elderly, skin traction — 2.25 kg (5 lb).
In the young and the middle aged, skeletal traction via a tibial traction pin.
Always measure the serum calcium preoperatively as hypercalcaemia is common.

Indications for surgery

Treatment
These fractures must be internally fixed unless the patient is moribund. Fixation may at least provide relief of pain and allow the patient to be nursed in bed without traction. At best, it allows immediate mobilization and thus a better quality of life.

Operation: internal fixation of pathological fractured shaft of femur

The implant used depends on the fracture, the surgeon and the devices available. Choices of implant include a variety of intramedullary nails which all have some sort of locking device. These include the Küntscher nail, Zickel nail, Reconstruction nail and Gamma nail. Alternatively, if the fracture looks as though it may be stable once fixed, a long nail-plate may suffice. The operative technique is the same as for non-pathological fractures, except that the fracture is exposed so that a specimen of bone can be taken for histology.

Codes
GA/LA . . . .   GA . . . .
Blood . . . .   4 units . . . .
Antibiotics . . . .   Yes . . . .
Time . . . .   1 ½ hours . . . .
Drains . . . .   Yes . . . .
Plaster . . . .   0 . . . .
Postoperative radiograph .   AP and lateral femur . . . . .
Stay . . . .   2 weeks . . . .
Follow up . . . .   6 weeks . . . .

**Operative
requirements**
Orthopaedic traction table.
Image intensifier and radiographer.

Postoperative care

Management
Mobilize the patient as soon as the pain allows. Referral to an oncologist should be made if the tumour is sensitive to radiotherapy. It is usually best to wait for the skin to heal before commencing radiotherapy.

Monitor the serum calcium, especially if the patient becomes confused or drowsy.

Complications
Beware multiple secondaries. Pain at the site of a known secondary often implies an impending fracture. This may benefit from prophylactic fixation.

Beware hypercalcaemia which can cause acute confusion and may be difficult to treat.

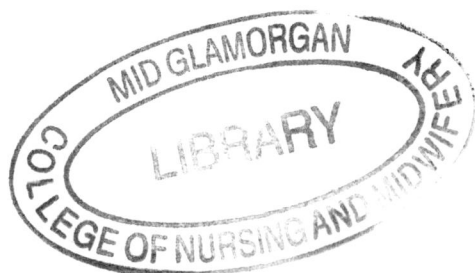

The condition
This fracture usually results from a fall onto a flexed knee.

Making the diagnosis

The patient

It mainly occurs in the middle aged and elderly.

On examination

There is usually a bruise at the site of impact.

If the fracture fragments are displaced, you should be able to feel a gap between them.

There may be some boggy swelling, but there is not normally a large haemarthrosis. This is because, with a displaced fracture, the quadriceps expansion is torn allowing the blood to disperse.

Examine the patient to see if they are able to extend the knee actively. This is best demonstrated by flexing the patent's knee passively and then asking them to lift their heel off the bed.

Active extension is lost with a displaced fracture of the patella.

Radiographs

AP and lateral views of the knee will show the fracture. Most fractures are transverse, but some are comminuted. If on the lateral view, the fragments are widely displaced, then the quadriceps expansion must be ruptured.

Make sure that what seems like an oblique fracture of the upper part of the patella is not in fact a bipartite patella. This is an ossification centre that remains separate from the rest of the patella and is generally present bilaterally. Therefore order a radiograph of the other knee to see if the uninjured patella is similar in appearance.

Preoperative management

Preparation for surgery

Whilst waiting for surgery, place the leg in a back-slab with the knee extended.

Treatment

An undisplaced fracture is treated conservatively, with the leg immobilized in a long leg cylinder for 6 weeks. Radiographs must be taken at 1 and 2 weeks to ensure that the fracture has not displaced.

If the fracture is displaced, continuity of the quadriceps mechanism must be restored. It is usually possible to reconstruct the patella if it is in only two or three fragments.

If it is a very comminuted fracture, the patella may have to be excised.

There may be one large fragment and several small ones. In this case, the small fragments are removed and the patellar tendon is wired to the remaining large proximal patellar fragment.

Indications for surgery

A fractured patella that is displaced.
Inability to straight-leg raise.

Operation: tension band wiring of fractured patella

The fracture is exposed through a midline incision. The fracture is reduced and then held with two parallel K-wires around which is passed a flexible wire. The ends of the flexible wire are twisted together. With this construct, flexion of the knee puts tension on the repair which is converted to compression of the fracture.

Codes

GA/LA	GA . . . .
Blood	0 . . . .
Antibiotics	Yes . . . .
Time	1 hour . . . .
Drains	Yes . . . .
Plaster	Back-slab . . . .
Postoperative radiograph .	AP and lateral knee . . . . . .
Stay	1 week . . . .
Follow up	6 weeks . . . .
Off work	6 weeks . . . .

Operative requirements	Wiring set. High thigh tourniquet.

Postoperative care

Management The knee is rested in a back-slab for 2 or 3 days. The patient is then mobilized, partially weight bearing between crutches, with or without a back-slab for support. Four or five days after surgery, when the wound is stable and if the fixation is sufficiently solid, active flexion and extension exercises can be started. The continuous passive motion (CPM) machine may then also be used.

Complications Inadequate fixation.
Wound breakdown.
Late osteoarthritis if imperfectly reduced.
Discomfort over the wires, necessitating their removal after the fracture has healed.

The condition

Osteoarthritis of the knee may be secondary to previous intra-articular trauma, meniscectomy, crystal arthropathy or simple obesity. The knee is commonly affected by rheumatoid arthritis.

Making the diagnosis

The patient

The patient is usually in their middle or old age. The elderly patient may have problems in other joints as well as medical problems. One has to ensure that giving them a pain-free knee will allow them greater mobility. For example, if their angina is so severe as to be the limiting factor in their activities, a knee replacement may be a waste of time as well as hazardous to their health.

The history

Ask about any previous knee problems or operations.

The most significant complaint is pain. Establish the following:

For how long can the patient walk before the pain makes them stop.

Whether the pain wakes them at night.

What analgesics the patient takes and how often.

Does the knee give way, swell or lock?

How does the patient go up stairs? Normally, or one stair at a time?

If the patient has rheumatoid arthritis, consider whether problems in other joints will limit their mobilization following surgery. Also try to ascertain whether the knee pain is worse than any hip pain that they may have.

On examination

Watch the patient walk. Note any limp and how a stick is used.

Look at the alignment of the leg. Is there a varus or valgus deformity when the patient is standing?

Look for scars from previous surgery to the knee (which the patient may omit to mention if many years previously).

Examine the knee to see if any swelling is due to osteophytes or an effusion or both.

Check the integrity of the collateral ligaments. If the medial collateral ligament is intact, a varus knee that is due to medial joint collapse can usually be brought straight and then an end point is felt. This is different to a knee that can be brought into varus due to laxity of the lateral collateral ligament.

Examine the range of flexion and extension, and in particular the presence of a flexion contracture and/or the inability to flex the knee beyond 90 degrees.

Do not omit to examine the movements of the hips and the neurological and vascular status of both limbs.

Note any signs of venous stasis that imply previous venous problems, especially a deep vein thrombosis.

If the patient has rheumatoid arthritis, examine all the major joints, especially the neck and temporomandibular joint.

Radiographs   Obtain recent AP and lateral radiographs of the knees. Ideally, one should obtain standing films of both legs. This allows estimation of the true varus/valgus deformity.

If the patient has rheumatoid arthritis, obtain views of the cervical spine.

Preoperative management

Investigations   Always obtain a midstream urine for microscopy, culture and sensitivity in a patient undergoing prosthetic replacement.

Treatment

The initial treatment for all arthritic joints is medical. This includes analgesics and anti-inflammatory drugs, as well as physiotherapy. The use of a walking stick and a non-steroidal anti-inflammatory drug may be enough to relieve the pain in many patients.

Indications for surgery

The primary aim of any surgery for arthritis is to relieve pain. Although there may be improved movement or stability, these are secondary benefits and not the reason for performing surgery.

A high tibial osteotomy may be performed for medial compartment osteoarthritis in the knee of a relatively young person (less than 60 years). The aim of the osteotomy is to correct deformity and shift some of the load away from the diseased part of the joint. Even a perfectly performed osteotomy cannot guarantee complete resolution of symptoms. In addition, if there is symptomatic improvement, although it may last for years, it will not last for ever. Most patients will need a total knee replacement in the future.

Degeneration that is confined to either the medial or the lateral compartment may be suitable for a unicondylar knee arthroplasty.

Joint destruction throughout the knee, accompanied by severe pain, is treated with a total knee replacement.

If a knee replacement becomes infected or loose, it is revised if at all possible. However, this is not always possible and the knee may have to be fused.

Contra-indications to surgery

Minimal symptoms, however severe the radiographic changes.

Severe flexion contracture.

Ischaemic heart disease or peripheral vascular disease which would obscure the benefits of knee replacement; i.e. if angina or claudication are so severe that the patient will not be able to walk very far following surgery, the risks may outweigh the benefits.

Urinary tract infection.

Prostatism that may result in postoperative urinary retention and the need for a prostatectomy. It is better to have the urological investigations and surgery *before* a knee replacement.

Operation: high tibial osteotomy

Using either a midline or transverse incision, an osteotomy is made in the upper tibia about 2.5 cm (1 in.)

below the joint. For medial compartment disease, a wedge of bone is removed that is laterally based. The gap is closed and the osteotomy is held with one or two staples. This is a very stable arrangement and the patient's knee can be mobilized out of plaster post-operatively. A CPM machine may be used initially after surgery. If a dome-shaped cut is made and the tibia realigned, the patient needs to stay in plaster whilst the osteotomy unites.

Codes

GA/LA	GA . . . .
Blood	2 units . . . .
Antibiotics	Yes . . . .
Time	1½ hours . . . .
Drains	Yes . . . .
Plaster	Yes . . . .
Postoperative radiograph	AP and lateral upper tibia . . . .
Stay	10 days . . . .
Follow up	6 weeks . . . .
Off work	3 months . . . .

Operative requirements

A high thigh tourniquet.

If the osteotomy is to be held with a staple, this should be specified on the operating list.

Management

Postoperative care

Measure the haemoglobin on the second postoperative day.

Mobilization depends on the exact method of fixation and the stability of the osteotomy.

Complications

Inadequate correction.

Loss of fixation and position.

Infection.

Deep vein thrombosis.

Persistent pain.

Operation: total knee replacement

The knee is opened via a midline skin incision and then the patella is reflected laterally. Using the guides supplied with each particular knee replacement, the surfaces of the femoral condyles, the tibial plateau and the patella are trimmed using a saw. The modern prostheses are essentially surface replacements and the minimum of bone is removed. The anterior cruciate is usually 'sacrificed'. The posterior cruciate ligament may or may not be retained, depending on the design of the knee replacement. The collateral ligaments are preserved as they are essential to the stability of these 'unconstrained' designs. The components articulate with each other, but are not linked.

The components of the knee replacement are usually cemented in place using bone cement but some prostheses are designed to be inserted without cement. Uncemented knee arthroplasty is preferable in the younger patient who is more likely to need revision surgery than an older patient.

Codes

GA/LA	GA . . . .
Blood	3 units . . . .
Antibiotics	Yes . . . .
Time	1½ hours . . . .
Drains	Yes . . . .
Plaster	0 . . . .
Postoperative radiograph . .	AP and lateral knee . . . . .
Deep vein thrombosis prophylaxis	According to consultant . .
Stay	10–14 days . . . .
Follow up	6 weeks . . . .
Off work	3 months . . . .

Operative requirements

The tourniquet has to be as high as possible on the thigh.

Management

Postoperative care

Unless the tourniquet was deflated prior to closure, knee replacements can drain up to 500 ml in the first few postoperative hours, so do not panic.

Check the foot pulses and sensation immediately after surgery.

Remove the drains after 24 hours.

Check the haemoglobin on postoperative day 2.

Mobilize the knee immediately, with or without the CPM machine.

The patient is allowed to begin walking, fully weight bearing, when he has good quadriceps control and is able to straight-leg raise.

Complications   Neuro-vascular injury.
Wound infection.
Deep vein thrombosis.
Deep infection of the prosthesis.
Late loosening.

Operation: revision of total knee replacement

Revision of a total knee replacement is considerably more difficult and hazardous than the primary operation.

If the revision is being performed for loosening, bony erosion has usually occurred that makes the fixation of the revision prosthesis more difficult. All the original cement has to be removed, but this is not as difficult as in a revision hip replacement. Special revision prostheses are used which are designed to compensate for the loss of bone and they usually have longer stems to aid fixation on both the femoral and the tibial components.

If the original prosthesis is being removed for infection, bone loss is usually less of a problem. The removal of cement, however, must be meticulous. The infected components are removed, but the new prosthesis is not inserted immediately. Instead, either beads or a spacer of antibiotic-impregnated cement are left in the wound. The patient is given the appropriate systemic antibiotic for 6 weeks. The knee is then reopened and the new components inserted.

Codes

GA/LA	GA . . . .
Blood	4 units . . . .
Antibiotics	Yes . . . .
Time	2 hours . . . .
Drains	Yes . . . .
Plaster	0 . . . .
Postoperative radiograph .	AP and lateral knee . . . . . .
Stay	3 weeks . . . .
Follow up	6 weeks . . . .
Off work	3 months . . . .

Operative requirements

High thigh tourniquet.

Management

Postoperative care

Remove the drains after 24 hours (n.b. they always drain a lot in the first few hours unless the tourniquet was deflated prior to closure).

Check the haemoglobin on postoperative day 2.

Many surgeons rest the knee extended in a back-slab, until the wound is stable. The knee is then mobilized with or without the CPM machine.

The patient is allowed to begin walking fully weight bearing, when he has good quadriceps control and is able to straight-leg raise.

Complications

Intraoperative fracture of femur or tibia.
Inability to insert new prosthesis.
Neuro-vascular injury.
Wound infection.
Deep infection of the prosthesis.
Deep vein thrombosis.
Late loosening.

Operation: arthrodesis of the knee

The knee is usually fused following failure of a total knee arthroplasty. The prosthesis is removed and the bone surfaces are cleaned of all debris and cement. If necessary, iliac crest bone graft is inserted into the gap to maximize the fusion rate. The knee is then held by one of two alternative methods. Either a stout intramedullary nail is passed from the femur into the tibia, or an external fixator is used.

Codes

GA/LA	GA . . . .
Blood	2 units . . . .
Antibiotics	Yes . . . .
Time	1 hour . . . .
Drains	Yes . . . .
Plaster	Only with external fixator . . . .
Postoperative radiograph	AP and lateral knee if external clamp used; AP and lateral femur and tibia if intramedullary nail used . . . .
Stay	2–3 weeks . . . .
Follow up	6 weeks . . . .
Off work	3 months . . . .

Operative requirements

If an intramedullary nail is to be used it must be long enough! Nails are available up to 700 mm in length.

If an external fixator is to be used, ensure that a complete set is available.

Postoperative care

Management

If an external fixator is used, an above-knee plaster may be needed for extra stability. Initially the patient must remain non-weight bearing. The transverse pins are removed after 6 weeks and a plaster cylinder is applied in which the patient can begin to weight bear. This plaster stays on for a further 6 weeks.

If an intramedullary nail is used, the patient can fully weight bear immediately.

Complications

Wound infection.

Failure to fuse.

Fracture of the tibia or femur at the tip of the nail.

Patello-femoral arthritis

The condition

Arthritis which mainly affects the patella is unusual, but can follow chondromalacia patellae or trauma.

Making the diagnosis

The history

The patient complains of a pain that is maximal behind the patella and worsens on walking up and down stairs.

On examination

The main finding of note, apart from the scars of previous operations, is the crepitus which is felt when you move the patella from side to side with a little downwards pressure. This is usually accompanied by pain.

Radiographs

Lateral and skyline views of the knee show a loss of joint space and osteophytes.

Treatment

Indications for surgery

Surgery is only warranted for severe degeneration of the articular surface of the patello-femoral joint that is accompanied by severe pain. The only option at present is to excise the patella.

Operation: excision of the patella

Either a transverse or a longitudinal midline skin incision is made. The patella is carefully shelled out whilst taking care to preserve the vertical fibres of the quadriceps. The continuity of the quadriceps expansion is thus maintained.

Codes
GA/LA .... GA ....
Blood .... Group and save ....
Antibiotics .... Yes ....
Time .... 1 hour ....
Drains .... Yes ....

Plaster .... Yes, cylinder ....

Postoperative radiograph . 0 ....

Stay .... 2 weeks ....

Follow up............. 6 weeks ....

Off work .... 3 months ....

**Operative
requirements**   High thigh tourniquet.

Postoperative care

Management   Static quadriceps exercises are started as soon as
possible.

The patient can be placed on CPM machine
immediately.

Walking is allowed when the patient is able to perform a
straight-leg raise, the pain has settled and the range
of motion is satisfactory.

Complications   Extension lag — the patient raises the leg in slight
flexion when trying to raise the leg straight.

Loss of full flexion.

59   Torn meniscus in the knee

The condition

This is a common injury. In lay terms, patients refer to having a torn cartilage. It is worth explaining (to the patient) that cartilage is actually the lining of the joint that covers the bone and that there are two menisci which are structures within the joint. This helps avoid confusion when a patient is told that the cartilage of the joint is intact but that a torn meniscus has been removed.

The medial meniscus is more commonly injured than the lateral.

A bucket handle tear is tear parallel to the free edge of the meniscus with the ends remaining intact. This 'bucket handle' can flip in and out of the middle of the joint and give rise to locking.

With a horizontal cleavage tear, the plane of the tear is parallel to the flat surface of the meniscus. It does not need to be removed.

A parrot beak tear is a split in either the anterior or posterior horn of the meniscus.

Making the diagnosis

The patient

Injury to the meniscus is very rare in children.

In young active adults, most symptomatic tears occur after a significant injury.

Less force is required to tear the meniscus in the older patient.

The history

In the young active adult, the meniscus is torn by a twisting injury to the flexed, weight-bearing knee. This may occur during games such as football, when the patient has all their weight on one leg with the knee bent and is twisting at the same time. Usually a sharp pain is felt in the knee, but it does not stop them from finishing their game. The knee swells over several hours, although not dramatically. If the patient is not treated and returns to sports, he may complain of pain over the medial or lateral joint line after activity.

191

The knee may lock. True locking occurs if the knee cannot be fully extended due to a mechanical block, but can be flexed almost fully. Without treatment, a knee may remain locked for days and then spontaneously unlock, often whilst the patient is asleep. You must distinguish this from what patients describe as locking. This is when pain in the knee prevents them from flexing the extended knee.

A more severe injury, such as a skiing accident, may result in 'the unhappy triad' — torn medial meniscus, torn anterior cruciate ligament and ruptured medial collateral ligament (see Chapter 60).

On examination   A full examination of the acutely injured knee is not possible since this causes too much discomfort. If the knee is not locked and there is not a huge effusion (which would suggest a ruptured anterior cruciate ligament), the knee is best examined after it has been rested for about 10 days.

Look for an effusion and quadriceps wasting.

Examine the range of movement of both knees. Many people normally have a degree of recurvatum; i.e. if you lift the heel off the couch, the knee may hyper-extend a few degrees. It is significant if this has been lost on the injured side.

Flex the knee and examine for tenderness along the joint line.

Perform McMurray's test. This is impossible to describe and is best demonstrated!

Check on the integrity of the anterior cruciate ligament by performing an anterior draw with the knee flexed at 90 degrees and with Lachmann's test with the knee flexed 10 degrees.

Examine the collateral ligaments.

Radiographs   Radiographs of the knee are normal.

Preoperative management

Investigations   Some surgeons like to confirm the clinical diagnosis of a meniscal tear with an arthrogram. Their aim is to reduce the number of arthroscopies performed on normal knees.

Common associated injuries

Torn anterior cruciate ligament and/or the medial collateral ligament.

Treatment

If there is a tense haemarthrosis or the knee is truly locked, the knee should be arthroscoped on the next convenient operating list to establish the source of the bleeding or the cause of the locking. A patient with a knee that repeatedly locks or gives way, should undergo an elective arthroscopy.

Indications for surgery

Presumed internal derangement of the knee, e.g. meniscal tear.

Prelude to further procedure, e.g. unicondylar knee replacement or anterior cruciate ligament reconstruction.

Contra-indications to surgery

Complete resolution of symptoms.

Operation: arthroscopy of the knee

Under a general anaesthetic, the knee is viewed using an arthroscope. This is a fibre-optic telescope that is approximately 5 mm wide and is inserted via a small stab incision. The whole of the inside of the knee joint can be inspected. Special instruments can be introduced into the knee via other small incisions. The arthroscope can be linked to a video camera so that the image is displayed on a television monitor for all to see. The camera allows an assistant to hold the arthroscope, leaving the surgeon free to operate with both hands.

If there is likely to be a torn meniscus, you must consent the patient for an arthroscopic partial meniscectomy, *plus* a possible open meniscectomy. Patients who have undergone an open procedure have a longer recovery period, both as an in-patient and as an out-patient.

Arthroscopy of the acutely injured knee is not easy. Extra care has to be taken if the collateral ligament is disrupted since the capsule will also be torn. This capsular tear allows the irrigation fluid to run out of the knee into the calf and may result in a compartment syndrome.

Codes

GA/LA	GA ....
Blood	0 ....
Antibiotics	0 ....
Time	¾ hour................
Drains	0 ....
Plaster	0 ....
Postoperative radiograph .	0 ....
Stay	Day-case ....
Follow up.............	1 week ....
Off work	Few days ....

Operative requirements

High thigh tourniquet.

Management

Postoperative care

If no procedure other than looking inside the knee is performed, the patient can go home the same or next day with crutches.

If an arthroscopic procedure (e.g. partial meniscectomy) is performed, this can still can be done as a day-case. However, the length of the procedure and anaesthetic may necessitate overnight admission.

Sometimes, due to difficulty in removing the meniscus arthroscopically, it is necessary to actually open the knee through a formal arthrotomy. If so, the patient has to remain in hospital until he can straight-leg raise and is able to walk.

Complications

Missed lesion, leading to persistent symptoms.
Infection.

60   Ruptured anterior cruciate ligament

The condition
Rupture of the anterior cruciate ligament is common. The patient may either be seen immediately following the injury or the diagnosis may be made when the patient complains of pain and instability weeks or months after the acute episode.

Making the diagnosis

The patient

The patient is usually a young adult who injures the knee whilst engaged in a sport such as skiing or football.

The history

The typical history is of a twisting injury to the knee with immediate pain. The gross swelling of the knee, which occurs within half an hour of the injury, is pathognomonic of either a torn anterior cruciate ligament or an intra-articular fracture. The patient is unable to continue the activity and hobbles off the football field or is carried off the ski slope.

If the patient is seen sometime after the acute episode, he complains of a feeling of instability that is most marked on going down stairs. The knee may swell and ache after sports. Locking is not typical of a ruptured anterior cruciate ligament. Remember, however, that the medial meniscus and the medial collateral ligament may be injured at the same time as the anterior cruciate ligament, as part of 'the unhappy triad'.

On examination

There is usually a haemarthrosis following rupture of the anterior cruciate ligament. This may remain for up to 2 weeks and the severe pain that accompanies the haemarthrosis prevents a complete examination of the knee.

In the examination of the non-acutely injured knee, the signs of a ruptured anterior cruciate are:
(a) a positive Lachmann's test;
(b) a positive anterior draw sign;
(c) a positive pivot shift.

195

Always examine the integrity of the collateral ligaments and perform a McMurray's test to examine the menisci.

Radiographs

If the bony origin of the anterior cruciate origin has been avulsed from the tibia, the bony fragment may be visible on radiographs of the knee. On the AP view, the fragment may be seen in the intercondylar notch and on the lateral view, it may lie just above the anterior tibial plateau.

A fluid level may be seen on the lateral view of the knee. This is due to a lipo-haemarthrosis.

Common associated injuries

Medial meniscus bucket handle tear.
Rupture of the medial collateral ligament.

Treatment

If a patient has a tense haemarthrosis and is not going directly to theatre, aspirate the joint using a full aseptic no-touch technique. This will provide great relief of pain as well as confirming the presence of blood in the knee.

Indications for surgery

Some surgeons like to take all patients with a haemarthrosis to theatre to wash out the joint, perform an arthroscopy and establish the exact diagnosis.

Augmentation procedures for complete rupture of the anterior cruciate ligament are indicated in a young adult with severe symptoms. The patient must be prepared to spend 6 weeks in a plaster with the knee flexed, followed by several months of postoperative physiotherapy and up to 6 months off work. The diagnosis of a ruptured anterior cruciate ligament must be confirmed at arthroscopy, prior to reconstruction/augmentation.

Operation: Jones's reconstruction of the anterior cruciate ligament; MacIntosh's antero-lateral stabilization of the knee

In the Jones's reconstruction of the anterior cruciate

ligament, the middle third of the patella tendon is removed with bone attached at either end. A hole is drilled in through the upper tibia and exits at the point of origin of the anterior cruciate ligament on the tibial plateau. The 'graft' is passed through this hole and round the back of the lateral femoral condyle, to the lateral side of the condyle where it is stapled into place. The aim is to replicate the path of the deficient ligament.

To provide extra lateral stability, a strip of fascia lata is detached proximally, passed under the lateral collateral ligament and around the intermuscular septum and sutured back on itself. This is the MacIntosh procedure.

Codes

GA/LA	GA . . . .
Blood	Group and save . . . .
Antibiotics	Yes . . . .
Time	1½ hours . . . .
Drains	Yes . . . .
Plaster	Above knee, with knee in 30 degrees of flexion . . .
Postoperative radiograph .	AP and lateral knee . . . . . .
Stay	5 days . . . .
Follow up	6 weeks . . . .
Off work	3 months minimum . . . . . .

Operative requirements

High thigh tourniquet.

Postoperative care

Management

The knee is immobilized in an above-knee cylinder, with the knee flexed approximately 30 degrees. This is kept on for 6 weeks. The patient is discharged from hospital once they are safe on crutches. Intensive physiotherapy is commenced once the plaster cast has been removed.

Complications

Neurovascular injury.
Compartment syndrome.
Lax reconstruction leading to persistent symptoms.
Permanent loss of full extension.

The condition

Chondromalacia means softening of the articular cartilage. The cartilage becomes soft, soggy and irregular. This can be due to a single injury to the cartilage. More commonly it is due to faulty tracking of the patella over the femoral condyle during flexion of the knee, which results in excessive pressure on the cartilage. The true nature of the condition is not known. Furthermore, why only the patellar side of the patello-femoral joint is affected, is not understood.

Making the diagnosis

The patient   This is a common problem in teenage girls, but not exclusively so.

The history   The patient complains of diffuse pain in the front of the knee without any specific injury. The knee does not truly lock or give way.

On examination   There may be a slight effusion. With the knee extended, palpate the articular surface of the patella, with the patella displaced medially and then laterally. There may be an area of tenderness.

Radiographs   Radiographs of the knee, although routinely ordered, are usually normal.

Treatment

The initial treatment is always conservative. The patient is advised to avoid excessive activity and to take a non-steroidal anti-inflammatory drug. If the problem persists, the knee can be arthroscoped to confirm the diagnosis. The soft area of cartilage can be curetted and drilled arthroscopically. This may give relief of pain that may or may not be permanent.

If the cause for the chondromalacia is excessive lateral pressure, a lateral release may be performed.

This is usually performed 'closed' through a small incision. The cutting of the lateral capsule can be seen with the arthroscope, but is often judged by feel alone.

Operation: lateral release of the knee

The aim of this procedure is to diminish the pressure on the lateral side of the patella by dividing the lateral capsule.

After an arthroscopy, a pair of scissors is inserted through a small skin incision, with one blade within the knee joint and the other outside the capsule (but under the skin). The scissors are run upwards, thus dividing the lateral capsule.

Codes

GA/LA	GA . . . .
Blood	0 . . . .
Antibiotics	0 . . . .
Time	15 minutes . . . .
Drains	0 . . . .
Plaster	0 . . . .
Postoperative radiograph .	0 . . . .
Stay	2 days . . . .
Follow up	2 weeks . . . .
Off work	2 weeks . . . .

Operative requirements

High thigh tourniquet.
Arthroscope.

Management

Postoperative care

A firm wool and crepe bandage is kept on for at least 48 hours as there is a risk of bleeding from the lateral geniculate vessels. If the knee is kept extended, the lateral structures that have been divided may repair themselves. Therefore the patient is either immediately placed on a CPM machine, or, if this is not available,

the knee is kept flexed at 90 degrees for 48 hours prior
to being mobilized.

Complications   Haemarthrosis.
Incomplete resolution of symptoms.

Cyst of the lateral mensicus

The condition

The true cause of cysts of the lateral meniscus is unknown. It has been suggested that they may develop as a sequel to previous trauma. The cyst may be associated with a tear of the lateral meniscus and the clinical features may be those of a meniscal tear. The neck of the cyst usually communicates with the knee joint.

Making the diagnosis

The patient

The patient is a young adult, more commonly male than female.

The history

The main complaint is of a bony hard lump on the lateral aspect of the knee. There may be an ache associated with the lump.

On examination

What the patient describes as a 'bony' lump is in fact a swelling on the antero-lateral joint line that is largest and hardest with the knee flexed to 90 degrees. With the leg fully extended the lump may disappear altogether.

Radiographs

Radiographs of the knee should be ordered, but are generally normal.

Treatment

Indications for surgery

A cyst that is painful and persists, can be excised surgically.

Operation: excision of a cyst of the lateral meniscus

Opinions vary on how best to remove these cysts. Some surgeons simply excise the cyst down to and into the joint. Some say that the knee should be arthroscoped and the cyst decompressed from within.

Most surgeons arthroscope the knee to ensure that there is no associated tear in the lateral meniscus. They then make an incision directly over the cyst and excise it.

Codes

GA/LA..................	GA ....
Blood	0 ....
Antibiotics	0 ....
Time...................	1 hour ....
Drains.................	0 ....
Plaster.................	0 ....
Postoperative radiograph ..	0 ....
Stay...................	3 days ....
Follow up	2 weeks ....
Off work	2 weeks ....

Operative requirements

Thigh tourniquet.
Arthroscopy equipment.

Postoperative care

Management

The patient is mobilized, fully weight bearing, when they are able to straight-leg raise.

Complications

Haemarthrosis from intra-articular bleeding.
Recurrence of the cyst.

63   Fracture of the tibial plateau

The condition
In the younger patient, this results from a high energy injury and may be one of multiple injuries. The fracture also occurs in elderly patients as the result of low energy trauma, such as a fall.

Making the diagnosis

On examination   The knee is usually very swollen and the leg may lie in valgus or varus. There may be a considerable haemarthrosis. Check the neuro-vascular integrity of the lower limb. If there is numbness in the leg or toes, this may be due to direct trauma to a nerve, commonly the lateral popliteal, or due to a developing compartment syndrome. Note the presence and location of any wounds or fracture blisters.

Radiographs   Order an AP and lateral views of the knee.
You may also need oblique views and/or AP and lateral tomograms or even CT scans to visualize the configuration of the fracture fragments.
The amount of depression of the articular surface has to be assessed since it is this that may require surgical correction.

Preoperative management

Preparation for surgery   Displaced fractures requiring surgery should be immobilized in a back-slab prior to going to theatre.
If massive swelling or fracture blisters prevent surgery being performed within 48 hours, it is best to place a tibial traction pin in the shaft of the tibia and place the limb on skeletal traction on a Braun frame. Four and a half kilograms (10 lb) of traction should be adequate.
If the patient is not having immediate surgery and there is a large haemarthrosis, it should be drained using a meticulous aseptic, no-touch technique. This will make the patient much more comfortable.

Treatment

The elderly patient with a minimally displaced fracture should be admitted. The limb is either immobilized in a plaster cylinder, or mobilized on the CPM machine. The choice depends on the patient and the availability of the equipment. The patient is mobilized by the physiotherapists after the pain settles.

Indications for surgery

A displaced fracture with depression of the joint surface.

Contra-indications to surgery

Compound injury or soft tissue injury over the line of the incision.

Operation: open reduction and internal fixation of tibial plateau fracture

The fracture fragments are exposed through a midline skin incision. The joint surface is elevated from below so as to restore the correct articulation. This creates a bony defect that has to be packed with bone graft. This may be taken from lower down the tibia, but is more commonly taken from an iliac crest. The fragments are held using buttress plates and screws.

Codes

GA/LA	GA
Blood	2 units
Antibiotics	Yes
Time	1–2 hours
Drains	Yes
Plaster	0
Postoperative radiograph	AP and lateral knee
Deep vein thrombosis prophylaxis	Yes
Stay	2 weeks
Follow up	6 weeks
Off work	3 months

Operative
requirements

Obtain consent for and include on the theatre list, the possibility of iliac crest bone graft.

High thigh tourniquet.

Standard AO set with buttress plates.

Postoperative care

Management

Remove the drains after 24 hours.

Beware compartment syndrome. If the patient has increasing pain unrelieved by splitting dressings *down to the skin*, call a more senior person — do not just give stronger analgesics.

If the surgeon is happy with the fixation, the patient may start mobilizing the knee immediately on the CPM machine. Otherwise the leg is immobilized in a plaster back-slab.

Patients need to remain non-weight bearing for 8 weeks.

Complications

Compartment syndrome.

Infection.

Deep vein thrombosis.

Loss of fixation.

Restricted range of movement.

Late osteoarthritis.

Making the diagnosis

The patient

This injury can occur at any age. Low velocity trauma produces simple, closed injuries. High energy injuries produce comminuted fractures that may be compound and may be accompanied by neurological or vascular damage. Unless the fracture is a result of a direct blow, always consider the patient to have suffered multiple trauma until proved otherwise.

The history

Establish exactly how the injury occurred. If the fracture is compound, in what environment did it occur? If it is a compound fracture, always inspect the covering garments. The lack of a hole in the trousers at the level of the fracture suggests that contamination is probably less than if the bone came through the trousers.

On examination

Look at the limb and at the state of the soft tissue over the fracture. Note the presence and location of any fracture blisters. A closed fracture can have such a severe soft tissue injury that the management is as difficult as if it were open.

If there is a wound that has been inspected and dressed, do not re-expose it. Each viewing increases the risk of infection.

Carefully examine the neurological and vascular status of the lower limb.

Examine the range of active and passive movement of the toes. If movement of the toes is accompanied by severe pain, consider compartment syndrome as a cause.

Radiographs

AP and lateral views of the whole tibia are essential. Make sure that both the knee and the ankle can be seen. If the original radiographs are obliques taken in the ambulance service's splint, ask for true AP and lateral views.

Common associated injuries

Preoperative management

Soft tissue trauma to lower leg.
Neuro-vascular injury.
Acute compartment syndrome.

Preparation for surgery

If the leg is grossly deformed, give the patient some analgesia and pull it straight. Do not wait for radiographs to confirm an obvious diagnosis.

Place the limb in an above-knee back-slab whilst awaiting primary treatment.

You may need to insert a calcaneal traction pin. This can be inserted in the accident department under local anaesthetic. Then arrange skeletal traction on a Braun frame with 4.5 kg (10 lb) of traction.

Treatment

An undisplaced fracture can be placed in a plaster cast immediately.

If the fracture is displaced, it may need to be reduced into an acceptable position. Once reduced the position may be maintained in a plaster cast, or internal fixation may be necessary.

Indications for surgery

An open fracture is a surgical emergency. Irrigation and debridement should be performed as soon as possible and certainly within 6 hours following the injury (not arrival in casualty). Once clean, the fracture is immobilized either in plaster, or in skeletal traction, or with an external fixator.

Most tibial fractures need some form of intervention, even if only a manipulation. The position is only acceptable if there is no varus/valgus angulation, no rotational deformity and the overlap of the shaft is 50% or more.

If the fracture is unstable or has failed a trial of conservative treatment, it may require internal fixation. This is either by an intramedullary nail or a plate.

As a rule, plates and nails are removed 18 months after their insertion.

Operation: manipulation under anaesthesia of a fractured shaft of tibia

Some fractures are easily manipulated into an anatomical position. Others can prove impossible to get bony apposition. This may be due to interposition of either tendon or muscle between the fracture ends. Once an acceptable reduction has been achieved, the next manoeuvre is to apply an above-knee plaster without losing the position.

There are several ways to reduce a tibia. You can manipulate the fracture with the lower leg hanging over the end of the operating table. Once reduced, you then put on the below-knee part of the plaster before extending the knee to continue the plaster above the knee. Alternatively, you can manipulate the leg with the knee extended and a block behind the knee, so that the below-knee part of the plaster can be applied. Once the plaster is set, move the block under the calf, and with the knee flexed at 15–20 degrees, continue the plaster above the knee.

Always split the plaster.

Codes

GA/LA	GA . . . .
Blood	0 . . . .
Antibiotics	0 . . . .
Time	½ hour . . . .
Drains	0 . . . .
Plaster	Above knee . . . .
Postoperative radiograph .	AP and lateral tibia . . . . . .
Stay	2 days . . . .
Follow up	1 week, X-ray on arrival . .
Off work	2–3 months . . . .

Operative requirements

Image intensifier and radiographer.

Radiolucent operating table.

The surgeon, plus an assistant who is skilled at applying plaster.

Management

Postoperative care

Beware *compartment syndrome*. If the patient has increasing pain unrelieved by splitting the cast down to the skin, call a more senior person — do not just give stronger analgesics. Reduced fractures should not hurt much!

Mobilize the patient non-weight bearing with crutches.

Children remain in plaster approximately 1 week for every year of their age, up to a maximum of 12 weeks.

Adults require a minimum of 12 weeks in plaster. The second 6 weeks can be in a below-knee, patella tendon-bearing (Sarmiento) cast, in which they can bear weight.

Complications

Compartment syndrome.
Deep vein thrombosis.
Fat embolism.
Loss of position.
Delayed union.
Malunion.
Non-union.

Operation: irrigation and debridement of open tibial fracture +/− insertion of calcaneal traction pin or application of external fixator

Under a general anaesthetic, the wound edges and all the injured tissue have to be excised and all dirt removed.

If a motorcyclist comes off at speed and suffers a compound tibial fracture, the proximal fragment may dig into the ground forcing dirt high up the medullary canal. One has therefore to deliver the ends of the fracture into the wound and ensure that the medullary canal is free of contamination.

It is best not to close compound wounds, however tempting.

Once the wound is clean, the fracture must be reduced and then immobilized. It may be possible to immobilize a stable fracture with a grade I wound in a long-leg plaster back-slab. All other compound tibial fractures are immobilized with either traction through a calcaneal traction pin or with an external fixator. The aim is to allow unimpeded access to the wound. The decision about which method to use depends on the wound, the surgeon and the apparatus available:

A calcaneal traction pin is generally inserted if the wound looks as though it may be possible for it to be closed when inspected after 48 hours. If the wound is clean, internal fixation may then be performed.

For most grade II and grade III fractures, an external fixator is applied with two pins above and two below the wound.

Codes

GA/LA	GA . . . .
Blood	4 units . . . .
Antibiotics	Yes . . . .
Time	1 hour . . . .
Drains	0 . . . .
Plaster	Yes, if not on traction . . . .
Postoperative radiograph .	AP and lateral tibia . . . . . .
Stay	10 days . . . .
Follow up	1 week . . . .
Off work	3 months . . . .

Operative requirements

Complete external fixator and pins.
Radiolucent operating table.
Image intensifier and radiographer.

Postoperative care

Management

Elevate the leg on a Braun frame.

Beware *compartment syndrome*. If the patient has increasing pain unrelieved by splitting the dressings down to the skin, call a more senior person — do not just give stronger analgesics. Remember that fractures that have been reduced should not hurt much!

Continue antibiotic cover for at least 48 hours.

Measure the haemoglobin on the first postoperative day.
Prepare the patient to return to theatre after 48 hours,
for inspection and further debridement if the wound
is still dirty, or wound closure and application of a
plaster cast or internal fixation if the wound is clean.

Complications
Infection.
Compartment syndrome.
Deep vein thrombosis.
Fat embolism.
Loss of position.
Malunion
Non-union.

Operation: intramedullary nail for fractured shaft of tibia

The nail is usually inserted 'closed'. That is to say that
the fracture itself is not opened and the nail is passed
across the fracture under radiological control.

With the patient on the orthopaedic traction table,
traction is applied via a calcaneal Steinmann pin and the
fracture is reduced. The incision goes either just to one
side or through the patella tendon. A guide wire is
passed down the medullary cavity, across the fracture.
Reamers are then passed over the guide wire to enlarge
the medullary cavity. The nail is then passed over the
guide wire.

An interlocking nail is usually used. These have cross
screws that go through both the bone and the nail, and
can be inserted proximally, or distally, or both. The use
of these locking screws depends on the level of the
fracture in relation to the isthmus. The isthmus is the
narrow mid-portion of the tibia. A fracture proximal to
the isthmus needs to be locked proximally as the nail
will only have a good grip in the distal fragment. A
fracture distal to the isthmus needs to be locked distally
as the nail will only have a good grip in the proximal
fragment. If the fracture is at the isthmus or is comminuted, the nail may require locking at both ends.

Codes

GA/LA	GA . . . .
Blood	2 units . . . .
Antibiotics	Yes . . . .
Time	1½ hours . . . .
Drains	Yes . . . .
Plaster	0 . . . .
Postoperative radiograph .	AP and lateral tibia . . . . . .
Stay	10 days . . . .
Follow up	2 weeks . . . .
Off work	6–12 weeks . . . .

Operative requirements

Image intensifier and radiographer.

Orthopaedic traction table.

A calcaneal traction pin is required, if not already *in situ*.

Management

Postoperative care

Elevate the leg on a Braun frame immediately post-operatively, prior to mobilization of the patient.

Beware *compartment syndrome*. If the patient has increasing pain, split the dressings down to the skin. If this does not relieve the pain, do not just give stronger analgesics, but call a senior person. Remember that reduced fractures should not hurt much!

When comfortable, the patient is mobilized either non-weight bearing or weight bearing, depending on the stability of the fracture fixation.

Complications

Infection.

Compartment syndrome.

Deep vein thrombosis.

Fat embolism.

Loss of position.

Non-union.

Operation: removal of tibial intramedullary nail

The end of the nail has to be found through the original incision and exposed clearly enough for the extraction device for that particular nail to be inserted. If the end of the nail is very deep, considerable excavation of the upper end of the tibia may be required. In addition, considerable force can sometimes be needed to extract the nail. In general it can be said that no one looks good taking out metalwork!

Codes

GA/LA................	GA ....
Blood	Group and save ....
Antibiotics	0 ....
Time.................	30–90 minutes.........
Drains................	Yes ....
Plaster................	0 ....
Postoperative radiograph ..	AP and lateral tibia......
Stay..................	2 days ....
Follow up	2 weeks ....
Off work	2 weeks ....

Operative requirements

To ensure that the correct instruments are available, theatres must know *exactly* what kind of nail is to be removed; Küntscher, Grosse–Kempf, AO, Richards, etc., and if there are locking screws to be removed. If in doubt, look at the previous operating note.
High thigh tourniquet.

Postoperative care

Management

Mobilize immediately, but keep the patient partial weight bearing for 2–3 weeks.

Complications

Refracture during nail removal.
Fracture not truly united.
Infection.
Compartment syndrome.
Refracture postoperatively.

65   Displaced fractures of the ankle

The condition
After fractures of the hip in the elderly, ankle fractures are the most common fractures requiring in-patient care. There are several classifications, none of which are universally accepted.

When assessing an ankle fracture you must consider whether there is injury to the malleoli, the medial and lateral ligaments or the interosseous membrane. Also consider the state of the soft tissues as this may determine the initial or even the definitive management.

Making the diagnosis

The patient

The patient may be of any age. In the young, prior to closure of the epiphyses, always remember that the ligaments are stronger than the epiphyses. In other words, children rarely have a ligamentous sprain. It is more likely that they have an epiphyseal injury and therefore must be X-rayed. In the elderly with osteoporotic bones, much less force is required to produce extremely comminuted fractures.

The history

Try to establish the exact mechanism of injury. Do not omit to ask where exactly the patient feels pain and always ask about pain along the whole length of the fibula.

Find out when the injury occurred, as fractures are ideally fixed within 6 hours of the event. After that time, soft tissue swelling may delay surgery until the swelling has subsided. This may take 6 days or more.

On examination

Examine for fibular neck tenderness, especially if there is medial malleolar pain but no lateral ankle pain. Palpate both sides of the ankle joint. Pain over the medial side without a medial malleolar fracture implies that there is a medial ligament injury.

214

Radiographs

The minimum requirement is an AP and lateral view of the ankle.

You have to see if the talus is displaced within the mortise or is likely to displace. If there is any doubt as to whether or not there is talar shift, ask for a mortise view (45 degrees internally rotated). Remember, however, that the talus is narrower posteriorly than anteriorly. This means that an AP radiograph with the foot in plantar flexion may appear to have a widened gap medially. If a back-slab is then applied with the foot at 90 degrees, the talus fills the mortise and the apparent shift is eliminated.

If there is talar shift and only a medial malleolar fracture, then the interosseous membrane must be disrupted and the fibula fractured more proximally. The fibular fracture may be as high as the fibular neck.

Preoperative management

Preparation for surgery

If the ankle is obviously dislocated — *reduce it*! The skin is at risk when the ankle is dislocated and prompt action can prevent a simple closed injury becoming open due to skin necrosis. Give the patient analgesics such as entonox and intravenous pethidine and simply correct the deformity. They will be far more comfortable once the dislocation has been reduced.

Immobilize all fractures in a back-slab, even if it is only a few hours before the patient will be operated upon.

Treatment

Undisplaced fractures of the ankle are immobilized in a plaster cast for 6 weeks.

If the fracture is displaced, it may be possible to manipulate the fracture into an acceptable position and then immobilize the fracture in a cast.

If the fracture cannot be manipulated into a satisfactory position or if the configuration is inherently unstable, open reduction and internal fixation is necessary. Since these fractures are intra-articular in a weight-bearing joint, the aim is to achieve a perfect reduction.

A very displaced fracture which needs open reduction

and internal fixation may be too swollen to operate upon immediately. It should be manipulated, placed in a back-slab and elevated until the soft tissue swelling diminishes.

Operation: manipulation under anaesthetic (MUA) of fractured ankle

The ankle is manipulated into as near an anatomical position as can be achieved and the position checked with either the image intensifier or plain films. Depending on the swelling around the ankle, apply either a well-padded back-slab or a full below-knee cast, that is immediately split.

Codes

GA/LA	GA
Blood	0
Antibiotics	0
Time	½ hour
Drains	0
Plaster	Below knee
Postoperative radiograph	AP and lateral ankle
Stay	4 days or until internally fixed
Follow up	1 week, X-ray on arrival
Off work	6 weeks

Operative requirements   Image intensifier and radiographer.

Management

Postoperative care

Elevate the leg on pillows or a Braun frame until the patient mobilizes.

If the reduction is acceptable and no further surgery is anticipated, the patient can be mobilized non-weight bearing with crutches.

The plaster can usually be completed prior to discharge.

The ankle is kept in a cast for 6 weeks.

Complications   Fracture blisters.
Loss of position.

Deep vein thrombosis.
Compartment syndrome.

Operation: open reduction and internal fixation (ORIF) of a fractured ankle

The medial malleolus is usually held by two parallel screws which are inserted near the tip of the malleolus and pass perpendicular to the fracture line.

The lateral malleolus is usually fixed using inter-fragmentary screws plus a plate. The exact arrangement depends on the configuration of the fracture.

Codes

GA/LA	GA ....
Blood	0 ....
Antibiotics	Yes ....
Time	1–2 hours ....
Drains	Yes ....
Plaster	Below-knee back-slab....
Postoperative radiograph .	AP and lateral ankle .....
Stay	7 days ....
Follow up.............	2 weeks ....
Off work	6 weeks ....

Operative requirements

Small fragment AO set.

Radiolucent operating table.

Plain films or image intensifier to check on the fixation.

A tourniquet is commonly used, but is in fact un-necessary if the leg is elevated in the Trendelenburg position during surgery.

Postoperative care

Management

Elevate the leg whilst the patient is in bed.

Remove the drains after 24 hours.

If the surgeon is happy with the fixation, active ankle movement out of the back-slab is commenced after 24 hours. When the patient can actively bring the ankle to 90 degrees, a full below-knee plaster can be applied. This early mobilization will mean that movement will be much better when the plaster comes off.

The patient remains in a cast for a total of 6 weeks. Two weeks non-weight bearing and then weight bearing for 4 weeks.

Complications

Wound breakdown.

Wound infection.

Compartment syndrome.

Deep vein thrombosis.

Loss of position if the fixation is inadequate or the bone is very osteoporotic.

Late osteoarthritis.

Operation: removal of internal fixation from the ankle

The screws and plates are removed through the original incisions. This is done in the young (less than 40 years), with a healed fracture, at least 18 months following internal fixation.

Codes

GA/LA . . . .   GA . . . .

Blood . . . .   0 . . . .

Antibiotics . . . .   0 . . . .

Time . . . .   1 hour . . . .

Drains . . . .   Optional . . . .

Plaster . . . .   0 . . . .

Postoperative radiograph .   AP and lateral ankle . . . . .

Stay . . . .   2 days . . . .

Follow up . . . .   2 weeks . . . .

Off work . . . .   2 weeks . . . .

Operative requirements

Tourniquet.

Theatre must know *exactly* what kind of metalwork is to be removed — whether small or large fragment AO. If in doubt look at the old operating note.

Management

Postoperative care
Mobilize the ankle immediately but keep the patient partial weight bearing for 2–3 weeks.

Complications

Poor wound healing.
Fracture not truly united.
Refracture postoperatively.

66   Arthritis of the ankle joint

The condition

Osteoarthritis of the ankle is unusual and may be the result of a fracture of the ankle or talus. Alternatively, it may be secondary to osteochondritis of the talus.

The ankle is commonly affected in rheumatoid arthritis.

Following a displaced ankle fracture, arthritis is unlikely to develop if the joint has been anatomically reconstructed. However, if the joint is not returned to a congruent state, secondary degeneration is very likely and will be evident 18 months following the injury.

Making the diagnosis

The history

The most important symptom to assess is pain:

Assess the severity and the frequency of the pain.

What medication is required to relieve the pain?

How far can the patient walk before stopping because of pain?

Does the patient walk with a stick?

Does pain from the ankle wake the patient at night?

On examination

Watch the patient walk. Do they limp? Do they use a stick?

Look for, and document, the position of any scars.

Examine the patient standing from behind and compare the alignment of the heels. Is the heel in valgus or varus?

Examine and compare the movements in both ankles. Be sure to separate the movements which occur in the ankle joint itself, from movement at the subtalar joint and the midtarsal joint. The movements of the ankle are best expressed as degrees of dorsi- and plantar flexion, whereas the subtalar and midfoot are best expressed as percentages of the normal.

Ensure that the pedal pulses are present and that sensation in the toes is normal.

Radiographs   AP and lateral views of the ankle are usually adequate.

Treatment

Indications for surgery   A painful ankle that is not improving, at least 18 months following the original injury.

Operation: arthrodesis of the ankle

This can be performed in a variety of ways. The ankle can either be approached medially, by detaching the medial malleolus, or anteriorly via a transverse or longitudinal incision. The articular surfaces of the tibia and the talus are denuded of cartilage and the surfaces made parallel.

Sometimes iliac crest bone graft is required to fill the gap between the bone surfaces.

The arthrodesis can be held with external compression clamps or with plates and screws.

Codes

GA/LA	GA ....
Blood	2 units ....
Antibiotics	Yes ....
Time	1½ hours ....
Drains	Yes ....
Plaster	Yes, below knee.........
Postoperative radiograph .	AP and lateral ankle .....
Stay	5 days................
Follow up.............	6 weeks ....
Off work	2–3 months...........

Operative requirements   Thigh tourniquet.

Compression clamp or AO plating set.

Consent for and include on the operating list, possible iliac crest bone graft.

Postoperative care

Management   Elevate the leg immediately postoperatively, and watch for compartment syndrome and wound problems.

Once the wound is stable, a below-knee plaster cast is applied and the patient mobilized non-weight bearing. After 6 weeks, the cast is changed to a weight-bearing cast. This is kept on until the ankle is clinically and radiologically united. This may take up to 14 weeks.

Complications   Neuro-vascular damage.
Poor position of fusion.
Failure of fusion.

67   Arthritis of the subtalar and midtarsal joints

The condition

These joints can be affected by rheumatoid arthritis. More commonly, previous fracture of the talus or the calcaneum can lead to secondary osteoarthritis.

Making the diagnosis

The history

The most important symptom to assess is pain:
Assess the severity and the frequency of the pain.
What medication is required to relieve the pain?
How far the patient can walk before stopping because of pain?
Does the patient use a walking stick?
Does the pain wake the patient at night?

On examination

Watch the patient walk. Do they limp? Do they use a stick?
Look for and document the position of any scars.
Examine the patient standing from behind and compare the alignment of the heels. Is the heel in valgus or varus?
Look for callosities from weight bearing in an abnormal fashion.
Compare the range of movements in both ankles and feet. Be sure to separate the movements that occur in the ankle joint itself, from movement at the subtalar joint and the midtarsal joint. The movements of the ankle are best expressed as degrees of dorsi- and plantar flexion, whereas the subtalar and mid-foot are best expressed as percentages of the normal. Also note which movements the patient finds painful.
Ensure that the pedal pulses are present and that sensation in the toes is normal.

Radiographs

Request AP and lateral views of the ankle and the foot.

Treatment

Indications for surgery

Arthrodesis of the tarsal joints is indicated either to stabilize and realign a paralysed foot or in the treatment of severe arthritis affecting the tarsal joints.

Operation: triple arthrodesis of the tarsal joints (combined subtalar and midtarsal arthrodesis)

The joints which are fused are the subtalar joint, the calcaneo-cuboid joint and the talo-navicular joint. This is done through a laterally based incision. The articular surface of the joints is removed and the bone surfaces apposed. If necessary, a wedge of bone is removed to correct a fixed deformity. The bones are usually held together using bone staples.

Codes

GA/LA	GA ....
Blood	Group and save ....
Antibiotics	Yes ....
Time	1 hour ....
Drains	0 ....
Plaster	Yes, below knee.........
Postoperative radiograph .	Whole foot ....
Stay	2 weeks ....
Follow up	6 weeks ....
Off work	2–3 months ....

Operative requirements

Tourniquet.
Bone staples.

Management

Postoperative care

Elevate the leg postoperatively until the patient is mobilized. The patient remains non-weight bearing between crutches for 5 weeks. After that time the patient is kept in a walking cast until there is clinical and radiological union.

Complications

Compartment syndrome.
Poor position of fusion.
Failure of fusion.
Continued pain despite radiological fusion.

The condition

This injury is common in the fourth and fifth decades. The rupture may be due to degeneration of the tendon.

Making the diagnosis

The patient

Typically the patient is a man in his early forties who has been playing an active sport such as squash or football.

The history

The patient will often describe the feeling that they had been struck on the back of the heel by their opponent's racquet (when they had not). They will have severe pain just above the heel.

On examination

With a complete rupture of the Achilles' tendon, there is bruising around the back of the heel and tenderness. There is usually a palpable gap between the ends of the ruptured tendon. The patient will not be able to stand on tiptoe.

Simmond's test is the definitive test for a ruptured Achilles' tendon. It is best performed with the patient kneeling on a chair. Squeeze the calf. This fails to produce plantar flexion of the foot if there is a complete rupture of the tendon.

Radiographs

A lateral view of the calcaneum should be taken to exclude avulsion of the tendon complete with a bony fragment. This is extremely rare.

Treatment

A complete tear that is seen within a few hours of the injury, may be treated conservatively in a plaster. Otherwise complete tears are repaired at operation.

Indications for surgery

A complete rupture of the tendo achillis.

Operation: repair of ruptured Achilles' tendon

A posterior longitudinal skin incision is made. Suture of the ruptured tendon is difficult, since the ends of the tendon are very ragged. Postoperatively, the repair is protected by placing the leg in a cast with the ankle plantar flexed.

Codes

GA/LA	GA ....
Blood	0 ....
Antibiotics	Optional ....
Time	1 hour ....
Drains	0 ....
Plaster	Below knee with the ankle plantar flexed ....
Postoperative radiograph .	0 ....
Stay	4 days ....
Follow up	2 weeks ....
Off work	6 weeks ....

Operative requirements

Tourniquet.

The operation is performed with the patient prone.

Postoperative care

Management

When comfortable, the patient is mobilized non-weight bearing.

The exact regime of out-patient care should be clearly stated by the surgeon in the operation notes, as there are several alternatives. A safe regime is:

(a) a below-knee cast with the ankle fully plantar flexed for 3 weeks;

(b) the cast is then changed to one with the ankle only partly plantar flexed, for 3 more weeks;

(c) once out of plaster, the patient should wear a shoe raise for 2 weeks.

The patient should only be allowed to play sport when he is able to stand on tiptoe.

Complications   Poor wound healing.
Wound infection.
Rerupture (approximately 10%).
Rupture of the other Achilles' tendon.

69   Fracture of the calcaneum

The condition
This fracture results from a fall where the patient lands on his feet. It is a common fracture and the long term result following a displaced fracture is often poor.

Making the diagnosis

The history
The patient will have fallen from a considerable height.
He will complain of pain in the heel and foot. He may have tried to weight bear but found it too painful.
It is important to ask about pain elsewhere, especially in the back.

On examination
Examine the foot and ankle with care. The common sign of a calcaneal injury is bruising in the instep of the foot that is like a thumb print. This is due to the spread of the haematoma being limited by the attachments of the plantar fascia. Compare the heels and note if the injured side has 'spread' relative to the normal.
Feel for tenderness over the spine, notably the thoraco-lumbar junction.

Radiographs
Order views of the calcaneum and the lumbar spine.

Preoperative management

Common associated injuries
Crush fracture of the first lumbar vertebra.

Treatment
Patients with a calcaneal fracture need to be admitted as they usually develop considerable swelling.
Place the leg in a below-knee back-slab with the ankle at 90 degrees. Elevate the leg on a Braun frame and instruct the nursing staff to apply regular ice packs.
The majority of calcaneal fractures are treated conservatively. Once the swelling has subsided, a below-knee plaster cast is applied and the patient is mobilized non-weight bearing with crutches.

Indications for surgery	There is considerable debate about the value of surgery. Due to the soft cancellous nature of the bone, manipulation of the fragments and insertion of screws is exceedingly difficult. However, a calcaneal fracture with depression of the subtalar joint, that is not comminuted, may be suitable for elevation of the joint surface and internal fixation.

Operation: open reduction and elevation of calcaneal fracture

The fracture is exposed through a lateral incision. The aim is to elevate the articular surface of the subtalar joint and then to pack in bone graft to help keep the joint surface elevated.

Codes

GA/LA	GA . . . .
Blood	Group and save . . . .
Antibiotics	Yes . . . .
Time	1 hour . . . .
Drains	0 . . . .
Plaster	Below knee . . . .
Postoperative radiograph .	Calcaneal views . . . .
Stay	1 week . . . .
Follow up	4 weeks . . . .
Off work	2–3 months . . . .

Operative requirements	Tourniquet. Obtain consent for, and include on the theatre list, the possibility of taking iliac crest bone graft.

Postoperative care

Management	Keep the leg elevated on pillows or a Braun frame until the patient is comfortable enough to mobilize. Then mobilize the patient non-weight bearing between crutches.

Complications	Wound infection. Subtalar arthritis.

70

Congenital talipes equino-varus — club foot

The condition

This is a common congenital foot deformity, occurring in males more often than females and is bilateral in one-third of cases.

The deformity is a combination of:

1 The talus pointing down and out — bringing the hind foot into equinus.

2 The navicular and the forefoot being shifted medially with additional supination — giving the varus deformity of the forefoot.

Making the diagnosis

The patient   The deformity is usually detected at birth.

On examination   Gently take the foot, bring it up and out and see if it can be brought into a normal position. If it can, the deformity is referred to as 'correctable'.

You must check for the associated conditions of spina bifida and arthrogryposis.

Radiographs   Radiographs in the newborn are not very helpful. Later, when the bones begin to ossify, the relationship of the talus to the calcaneum is measured on the AP and lateral views of the foot.

Treatment

Treatment must begin on presentation, with strapping of the foot in as near a corrected position as possible. This is applied without an anaesthetic and is replaced weekly. If at 6 weeks a full correction has not been achieved, operative correction is necessary.

Operation: postero-medial release for club foot

The aim is to divide or elongate any structures on the medial and posterior part of the foot which are preventing the foot from assuming a normal position.

This may include elongation of the tendo achillis, the tendons of tibialis posterior, flexor digitorum longus and flexor hallucis longus, and division of the capsule of the subtalar, talo-navicular and calcaneo-cuboid joints.

At the end of the operation, it should be possible to bring the foot into a normal attitude.

Codes

GA/LA	GA ....
Blood	0 ....
Antibiotics	0 ....
Time	1½ hours ....
Drains	0 ....
Plaster	Above knee, for 6 weeks ..
Postoperative radiograph .	0 ....
Stay	4 days ....
Follow up	2 weeks ....

Operative requirements

Paediatric tourniquet.

Management

Postoperative care

After 2 weeks, when the wound is healed, the definitive plaster is applied with the foot in the fully corrected position. The foot is kept in a plaster cast for 6 weeks.

Following removal of the plaster, the child wears special splints (Denis Browne boots) to prevent the deformity recurring. Splintage usually continues until the age of one.

Complications

Injury to the posterior tibial neuro-vascular bundle.
Wound breakdown.
Incomplete correction of the deformity.
Recurrence of the deformity.

71

Clawed toes

The condition
In children, clawing of the toes may be idiopathic or secondary to a neurological disorder. In an adult, the deformity may occur in an otherwise normal foot, or with a hallux valgus, or as a result of rheumatoid arthritis.

Making the diagnosis
The history The patient will complain of pain under the ball of the foot and callosities. The prominent proximal interphalangeal joints may also be sore. The patient will be unable to find a comfortable pair of shoes.

On examination In claw toes, the metatarsal phalangeal joints are hyperextended and are often subluxed or dislocated. The proximal and the distal interphalangeal joints are held flexed.

There may be callosities underneath the metatarsal heads and on the dorsum of the prominent proximal interphalangeal joint of the toes.

Check upon the neuro-vascular status of the foot, in particular the presence or absence of foot pulses.

Examine the back of a child who has claw toes, for a dimple or hairy patch that may indicate spina bifida occulta.

Radiographs Radiographs of the foot should be taken to exclude any other cause for pain. Look to see if any of the metatarsophalangeal joints are dislocated.

Treatment
Indications for surgery If the toes can be passively straightened, a dynamic correction can be performed to realign the toes (Girdlestone's procedure).

If the deformity is fixed (cannot be passively corrected)

but the metatarsophalangeal joints are *not* dislocated, (Helal's) metatarsal osteotomies are performed.

For a severe fixed deformity, where the meta-tarsophalangeal joints *are* dislocated, a forefoot arthroplasty is performed.

Operation: flexor to extensor transfer of toes (Girdlestone's procedure)

The long flexor of each toe is transferred into the extensor expansion over the dorsum of the proximal phalanx. This is done through lateral incisions on the second, third and fourth toes.

Codes

GA/LA	GA . . . .
Blood	0 . . . .
Antibiotics	0 . . . .
Time	45 minutes . . . .
Drains	0 . . . .
Plaster	0 . . . .
Postoperative radiograph .	0 . . . .
Stay	3 days . . . .
Follow up	2 weeks . . . .
Off work	6 weeks . . . .

Operative requirements

Tourniquet.

Management

Postoperative care

The toes may be held straight by strips of plaster of Paris on the dorsum of the toe. If used, these are kept on for 2 weeks.

The patient is mobilized fully weight bearing, as soon as the pain allows.

Complications

Inadequate correction.

Operation: dorsal displacement osteotomy of the metatarsal shafts (Helal's osteotomies)

A longitudinal dorsal incision is made between adjacent metatarsals so that the two can be operated upon through a single incision. The metatarsal necks are divided obliquely so that the metatarsal heads slide proximally and dorsally. No internal fixation is required. As a result the metatarsal heads are less prominent and the shortening of the metatarsal reduces the clawing of the toe.

Codes

GA/LA	GA ....
Blood	0 ....
Antibiotics	0 ....
Time	½ hour ....
Drains	0 ....
Plaster	0 ....
Postoperative radiograph .	AP and lateral forefoot ...
Stay	1 week ....
Follow up..............	2 weeks ....
Off work	6–10 weeks ....

Operative requirements   Tourniquet.

Management

Postoperative care
Mobilize after 2–3 days, heel walking.
When the pain subsides, the patient should be encouraged to weight bear on the front of the foot, otherwise the metatarsal heads may fall back into their original position.

Complications   Division of both neuro-vascular bundles to a toe.
Poor position of osteotomy.
Non-union.

Operation: forefoot arthroplasty (Kates–Kessel and Fowler's procedure)

In a simple (Kates–Kessel) forefoot arthroplasty, only the distal ends of the metatarsals are excised. This removes the prominent metatarsal heads and the resultant shortening of the toes relaxes the clawing. This procedure is performed through three separate longitudinal dorsal incisions.

In a Fowler's procedure, the bases of the proximal phalanges as well as the distal ends of the metatarsals are excised — in other words it is an excision arthroplasty of the metatarsophalangeal joints. In addition, an ellipse of plantar skin can be excised to draw back the anteriorly displaced pad of weight-bearing skin into its correct position.

Since both procedures shorten the foot, it should be performed on both feet and not on a single foot.

Codes

GA/LA	GA . . . .
Blood	0 . . . .
Antibiotics	Optional . . . .
Time	1 hour . . . .
Drains	0 . . . .
Plaster	0 . . . .
Postoperative radiograph .	AP feet . . . .
Stay	2 weeks . . . .
Follow up	6 weeks . . . .
Off work	3 months . . . .

Operative requirements

Tourniquet.
Powered saw.

Management

Postoperative care
Elevate the feet and keep the patient non-weight bearing until the wounds have healed.
Once the wounds are stable, the patient can mobilize full weight bearing as the pain allows.

Complications   Injury to the neuro-vascular supply to a digit, leading to
loss of a toe. This is a greater risk with the Fowler's
procedure.
Wound infection.
Persistent pain.
Slow recovery.

72   Hammer toe

The condition
This common condition is of unknown aetiology and commonly affects the second toe.

Making the diagnosis

The history
The patient complains of soreness over the proximal interphalangeal joint of the toe, unrelieved by propriety pads and plasters.

On examination
A hammer toe is a fixed deformity (cannot be passively corrected) and is equivalent to a boutonnière deformity in the finger — the metatarsophalangeal and distal interphalangeal joints are hyperextended whilst the proximal interphalangeal joint is flexed and thus prominent.

Treatment

Indications for surgery
Painful hammer toe.

Operation: fusion of the proximal interphalangeal joint for hammer toe

The extensor tendon is divided and the joint excised through an incision over the dorsum of the proximal interphalangeal joint. The toe may be held with a K-wire which is brought out through the end of the toe. If used, the wire is removed in the clinic after 6 weeks.

Codes
GA/LA . . . .   GA . . . .
Blood . . . .   0 . . . .
Antibiotics . . . .   0 . . . .
Time . . . .   ½ hour . . . .
Drains . . . .   0 . . . .
Plaster . . . .   0 . . . .
Postoperative radiograph .   0 . . . .

Stay .... 24 hours if a single toe ...
Follow up.............. 2 weeks ....
Off work .... 6−8 weeks ....

Operative
requirements

Tourniquet.
K-wire set and driver.

Postoperative care

Management

Check to see that the toe becomes pink once the tourniquet has been deflated. If the toe remains dusky, this may be due either to the vessels being stretched or the dressings being too tight. Push the end of the toe down the K-wire to reduce possible stretching of the vessels and release the dressings around the toe.

If only one toe is fused, the patient is able to mobilize with little discomfort. If multiple toes are fused, the patient may be able to be discharged after 1 or 2 nights, but should rest at home with the feet elevated until they feel comfortable enough to walk upon.

The wire is removed after 6 weeks, in the clinic.

Complications

Non-union of fusion.
Division of both neuro-vascular bundles to a digit.

The condition

The metatarsal of the big toe is displaced towards the other foot and the toe is angled away from the midline of the body and thus is in valgus. The condition may be familial or it may be acquired.

Making the diagnosis

The patient   The patient is usually a middle-aged female, although if the problem is congenital, it may present in the second or third decade.

The history   The main complaints are of a painful prominence over the medial side of the metatarsophalangeal joint and a widened foot that makes buying shoes difficult. If there is an adventitial bursa, this may become inflamed and give episodes of pain. There may be a family history of the condition.

On examination   The metatarsophalangeal joint is prominent and there may be a painful bursa over the joint. The great toe may be so angulated as to be pressing on or under the second toe.

Examine the great toe and see if it can be brought into a normal position.

Examine the range of flexion and extension of the metatarsophalangeal joint. If the joint is stiff, the pain may be due to osteoarthritis rather than hallux valgus.

Always check on the neurovascular status of the foot, especially if the patient is a diabetic.

Radiographs   Standing AP and lateral radiographs of the foot will show the deformity. In the elderly, the presence of degenerative changes in the metatarsophalangeal joint must be assessed.

Treatment

Indications for surgery

Deformity itself is not a reason to operate, however unsightly. Surgery is only indicated if the patient has persistent pain.

There are many different operations for hallux valgus:

In a patient under 70 years, without arthritis of the metatarsophalangeal joint, most surgeons perform some type of metatarsal osteotomy. The choice of osteotomy partly depends on the degree of valgus:

(a) if the valgus at the metatarsophalangeal joint is less than 30 degrees on the standing radiograph and is fully correctable on examination, a displacement osteotomy is adequate, e.g. chevron osteotomy;

(b) if the valgus is greater than 30 degrees, the metatarsal osteotomy should include a closing wedge to gain additional correction, e.g. Hohmann's osteotomy.

In a patient over 70 years, the simplest operation is to remove the proximal third of the proximal phalanx (Keller's excision arthroplasty) and the bony prominence.

Operation: chevron metatarsal osteotomy

A dorso-medial incision is made, centred over the first metatarsophalangeal joint. The bony prominence of the bunion is removed. An osteotomy is performed that displaces the metatarsal shaft laterally (towards the second toe) without any angulation. Because of its design (like the letter V on its side with the tip pointing distally), the osteotomy is very stable.

Codes

GA/LA	GA
Blood	0
Antibiotics	Optional
Time	½ hour
Drains	0
Plaster	Plaster slipper
Postoperative radiograph	AP and lateral great toe

Stay	3–4 days	
Follow up	3 weeks	
Off work	6 weeks	

Operative requirements

Tourniquet.
Fine power saw.

Postoperative care

Management

Elevate the foot until the patient is comfortable enough to mobilize. The patient can then walk heel bearing.

The plaster slipper is removed and the patient can weight bear on the whole foot after 3 weeks.

Complications

Wound infection.
Loss of position of osteotomy.
Non-union.
Persistent pain.
Avascular necrosis of the metatarsal head.

Operation: Hohmann's metatarsal osteotomy

A wedge of bone is removed from the neck of the metatarsal through an incision on the dorso-medial aspect of the joint. A peg is made on the proximal fragment, the distal fragment is displaced laterally and the two fragments impacted together. The medial capsule is reefed to help hold the toe straight and a K-wire can be used to hold the osteotomy.

Codes

GA/LA	GA	
Blood	0	
Antibiotics	0	
Time	½ hour	
Drains	0	
Plaster	Yes, if K-wire not used	
Postoperative radiograph	AP and lateral great toe	
Stay	2 days	
Follow up	2 weeks	
Off work	6 weeks	

Operative requirements

Tourniquet.

Power saw, drill and K-wire (if required).

Postoperative care

Management

Elevate the leg initially.

Mobilize the patient heel bearing when she is comfortable. The sutures are removed after 2 weeks and the wire is removed as a day-case under a brief GA after 6 weeks.

If no internal fixation is used, the plaster is changed after 2 weeks to a plaster slipper in which the patient remains for 4 more weeks.

Complications

Non-union.

Poor position of fusion.

Metatarsalgia under the metatarsal heads of the second to fifth toes.

Operation: Keller's excision arthroplasty

The joint is exposed through a dorso-medial incision. The bony prominence under the bunion and the proximal half of the proximal phalanx are removed. When it has healed, the great toe is shorter and is a little floppy.

Codes

GA/LA	GA
Blood	0
Antibiotics	0
Time	½ hour
Drains	0
Plaster	0
Postoperative radiograph	(Optional) AP and lateral toe
Stay	2 days
Follow up	2 weeks
Off work	6 weeks

Operative requirements

Tourniquet.

Management

Postoperative care

Elevate the leg initially.

Allow the patient to weight bear as the pain allows.

Complications   Too generous a resection of the proximal phalanx.

The condition
Metatarsalgia is pain under the metatarsal head. It may be due to a neuroma of one of the plantar digital nerves — a Morton's neuroma.

Making the diagnosis
The patient

Although it can occur at any age, this condition usually presents over the age of 40. It is more common in women.

The history

The patient will complain of extreme pain under the ball of the foot when weight bearing. She may describe the pain as feeling like she is walking on broken glass. The patient may have noticed some abnormal sensation in the toe supplied by the nerve.

On examination

On lateral compression of the metatarsal heads you may be able to elicit a palpable clunk that is accompanied by pain. Do not forget to examine the sensation in the toes.

Radiographs

Obtain radiographs of the foot to exclude any bony cause for the pain.

Preoperative management
Preparation for surgery

On the consent form, describe the operation exactly, e.g. excision of the digital nerve to the cleft of 4th/5th toes.

Clearly mark the affected cleft preoperatively on both the dorsum and plantar surfaces of the foot.

Warn the patient that the toes that are involved may be permanently numb following surgery.

Treatment
Indications for surgery

Symptoms and signs of a digital neuroma that has not responded to conservative treatment with pads, etc.

Operation: excision of plantar digital neuroma for Morton's metatarsalgia

The digital nerve is exposed through either a plantar or a dorsal longitudinal incision centred on the correct interspace. The common digital nerve (i.e. before it divides into two separate digital nerves) is located and is usually visibly enlarged. The nerve is excised. Due to the excision of the nerve, the toe web may be permanently anaesthetic after surgery, but pain free.

Codes

GA/LA	GA ....
Blood	0 ....
Antibiotics	0 ....
Time	30 minutes ....
Drains	0 ....
Plaster	0 ....
Postoperative radiograph .	0 ....
Stay	2–3 days ....
Follow up..............	2 weeks ....
Off work	3–6 weeks ....

Operative requirements

Tourniquet.

Send the resected nerve to histology to confirm that a nerve was resected and there was a neuroma. (This is very useful should the operation not be a success!)

Management

Postoperative care

Elevate the leg, before allowing the patient to mobilize on the first postoperative day.

Complications

Wrong diagnosis, leading to persistence of symptoms.
Tender scar.

The condition

This is remarkably common injury. The foreign body is often a needle or pin.

Making the diagnosis

The history

The patient usually presents on the day of injury, pretty certain that they have stepped on 'something' and complaining of pain in the foot.

On examination

There may be a puncture hole where the foreign body entered. If the injury occurred several days previously, look for signs of cellulitis or abscess formation.

Radiographs

Ask for radiographs of the foot in two planes, with a marker taped to the skin to indicate the entry hole. You will be surprised how far away the foreign body may be from its entry point.

Treatment

Unless you can actually see the end of the pin/needle, do not attempt to remove it in casualty under local anaesthesia. It can literally be like looking for a needle in a hay-stack and is often difficult for the surgeon and painful for the patient.

Indications for surgery

Any foreign body in the foot which is causing pain.

Operation: removal of foreign body from the foot

This is often a trickier procedure than you might expect. With the patient prone, the foreign body is visualized on the image intensifier. Two hypodermic needles should be inserted into the sole of the foot at right angles to each other, to establish the position of the object. A cut is made and then the object is located by a combination of screening with the image intensifier and feeling with an artery clip.

Codes

GA/LA	GA	
Blood	0	
Antibiotics	Yes	
Time	½–1 hour	
Drains	0	
Plaster	0	
Postoperative radiograph	0	
Stay	2 nights	
Follow up	2 weeks	
Off work	2 weeks	

Operative requirements

Tourniquet.
Image intensifier and radiographer.

Postoperative care

Management

The patient may weight bear immediately, as the pain allows.

Complications

Inability to retrieve the foreign body.
Wound infection.

Glossary

AO. Association for Osteosynthesis. This refers to the system of fracture fixation originated by the Swiss.

AO mini-fragment set. Set of plates and screws suitable for fixing fractures in the hand.

AO small fragment set. Set of plates and screws suitable for fixing forearm and ankle fractures.

AO standard fragment set. Set of plates and screws suitable for fixing large adult bones.

Arthrodesis. Surgical fusion of a joint.

Arthroplasty. An operation that restores function to a joint. This is commonly by replacement with an artificial joint, but not always. Excision of the joint without replacement is also an arthroplasty.

Calcar. The calcar is the relatively strong medial neck of the femur above the level of the lesser trochanter.

Closed (fracture). A fracture without an associated skin defect.

Comminuted. A term used to describe a fracture where the bone is in many pieces.

Compound (fracture). A fracture associated with a skin wound. Also referred to as an open fracture.

CPM (continuous passive motion). The CPM machine is a machine which flexes and extends a limb passively. The range and the rate of movement are adjustable.

Denham pin. A traction 'pin' that is up to 20 cm long and 5 mm in diameter. It is threaded in the middle third to prevent it sliding out of the bone.

Image intensifier. A X-ray machine that produces an instant image on a television monitor.

Kirschner wire, K-wire. A sharp stout 'pin' that may be between 10 and 20 cm long, and of various widths from 1.5 to 3 mm. It is inserted either using a hand-held chuck or with a powered K-wire driver.

Küntscher nail, K-nail. A long steel nail, used for the intramedullary fixation of fractures.

MUA. Manipulation under anaesthesia.

ORIF. Open reduction and internal fixation (of a fracture).

Osteotomy. A general term for surgical division of a bone.

Patella, patellar. Patella is the bone itself. Patellar is the adjective that refers to the bone.

Radiculogram. The radiological study of the spinal nerve roots and their sheaths after the injection of a radio-opaque contrast medium, which is water soluble.

Revision. In reference to operations, a revision is a second operation of the same nature as the first.

Steinmann pin. A traction 'pin' that is up to 20 cm long and 5 mm in diameter. It is smooth throughout.

TED. Thromboembolic deterrent (stocking).

Tomogram. A radiograph produced by tomography, where each image is of one layer of the body at any required depth.

Ulna, ulnar. Ulna is the bone itself. Ulnar is the adjective referring to the ulna (on the ulnar side . . .).

Volar. A synonym for palmar or plantar.

Index